DEDICATION
For those women who have come to a cross road in their life
where health and wellness are the foundation to beauty
and hair is simply its' reflection.

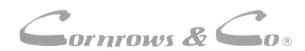

Cornrows & Co.®

Publication

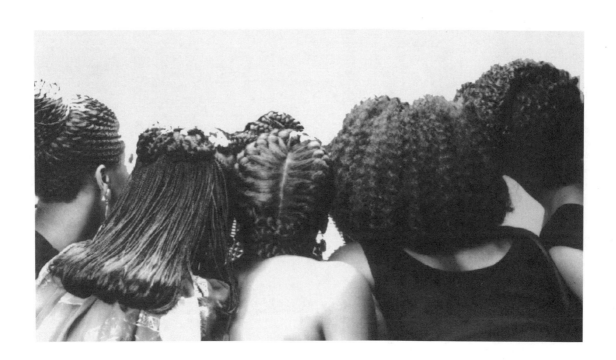

LET'S TALK HAIR

Every Black Woman's Personal Consultation
for Healthy Growing Hair

Pamela Ferrell

Foreword by A'Lelia Perry Bundles,
great-great granddaughter of Madam C. J. Walker

Published by Cornrows & Co. ®
Washington, DC

Published by Cornrows & Co.® Inc.
5401 Fourteenth Street NW
Washington DC 20011

Editor: Lurma Rackley
Art Director: Pamela Ferrell
Cover Photograph: Andre Richardson

10 9 8 7 6 5 4 3 2 1

Library of Congress Catalog Card Number 96-85919
Let's Talk Hair / Pamela Ferrell
ISBN 0-939183-02-1

Table of Contents

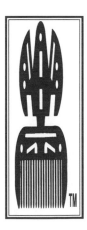

ACKNOWLEDGMENTS

To my clients and models who so patiently smiled to the camera after the long photo sessions, I am grateful for your participation.

Husband Taalib-Din, Love and thanks for your support and protection......I can always rely on you as a business partner...can't do this alone.

Baby Girl Amber, you have taught me that I must take a peanut butter and jelly sandwich break with you or I will not get any work done.

Senator Carol Moseley Braun, thank you for your wisdom and insight. You always leave me with the answers I didn't know I was seeking.

Diana Ross, I am ever more grateful for the invitation to the beach house. A writer's dream is to get away and peacefully write!

D'Michelle Berryman, thank you for the precious memories. You leave me with the reality that we must take responsibility for our health and never take it for granted.......I miss you dearly.

A special thanks to my audience of women who remind me at the most tiring times that hair care information for black women is needed.

AUTHOR'S NOTE

No matter where you go in the world, everyone has hair. Whether it is long, short, coily, straight, healthy or damaged, hair is the one topic that can cause people to dialogue, as well as exchange anecdotes about their personal hair experiences.

That is why I wrote this book, to share some secrets and guidance to make the whole idea of hair a healthy, uplifting and human experience. I once took for granted that women could easily access natural hair care tips in consultation with their hair braiders and hair stylists. Mistakenly, I assumed that most African-American women knew how to care for their natural hair; however, I discovered that is not the case. In <u>Let's Talk Hair</u> I have created for you a personal consultation with real answers to your hair questions and concerns.

My approach is a contradiction to modern cosmetology that promotes the use of harmful and toxic hair cosmetics for beauty, an industry that has side tracked into prettiness above your health and wellness. Like the wholistic healer up against the medical industry, a natural hair care advocate threatens the livelihood and false belief system that the chemical stylist promotes. My years of dedication and practice in natural hair care have well documented the profound fact that natural methods are safer, smarter and healthier for you. The powerful effects have caused a healing to my client's physiological, spiritual and mental wellness.

The cosmetology industry is recognizing that in order to prosper and stay current, they too must incorporate more natural methodology to their practice. To change their arrogant philosophy about African-American coily hair, however, would take more time and effort than I have to spare in this lifetime; so I will pass the information on to you since you stand to gain the most from it. I hope to take the mystery out of growing healthy hair and empower you with the insight and tools to self diagnose and remedy the simplest of hair care problems.

<u>Let's Talk Hair</u> is an attempt to respond to the backlash, misery and pain the African-American woman perpetually endures over her natural coily hair. It attempts to dig deep in the psyche and find answers that are in your mental lost and found department. My approach is basic, simple, honest and natural. Once you learn how to care for your natural hair, I hope you will have an exciting new image of yourself and feel touched to pass it on so that the ideal of healthy natural hair becomes contagious.

Pamela Ferrell

FOREWORD

A'Lelia Perry Bundles

Great great grand-daughter of Madame CJ Walker

Touch your hair. Weave your fingers deep into your roots and massage your scalp. Let all that pent-up tension evaporate. Now grasp a fistful of hair and twist it slowly around and around your fingers. Is it thick and springy? Wispy and limp? Crunchy? Cottony? Wavy? Wiry? Like straw? Like fleece? Do you love what you feel?

If hair designer and author Pamela Ferrell had her way--if she could wave a magic wand--we would all answer, "Yes!" We would all love our locks, and bad hair days would lose their meaning. We would get over this good hair/bad hair thang. We would be secure and confident and healed from the childhood traumas that little black girls feel when it's time to get their hair "done."

Pamela is probably the first to admit that she has no magic wand. But her deep concern, nurturing spirit and artist's touch provide the next best thing for unraveling the knots we've tangled around our psyches because of this mass of protein on our heads.

Long before I met Pamela I knew about her successful crusade on behalf of hair braiders in the District of Columbia when the local cosmetology board at first refused their right to braid. From afar I had admired Pamela and her husband Taalib-Din Uqdah for having the courage to challenge the status quo. As co-owners of Cornrows & Co. -- the nation's premiere natural hair care salon--they have testified in hearings and helped finance law suits against corporate giants whose cultural chauvinism led to no-braid policies in the workplace.

I marveled at the intricate, ancestor-affirming braids and twists Pamela conjured for the movie, "Daughters of the Dust". And I delighted in her knack for adapting traditional African hairstyles to African American hair-statements appropriate for corporate board-rooms and the halls of Congress.

Having grown up in a household where hair care was the family business, I have always had more than a passing interest in the value placed on hair in our community. My great-great-grandmother, Madam C. J. Walker--who, by the way, did not invent the straightening comb--was one of the pioneers of the modern black hair care industry. My late mother, A'Lelia Mae Perry Bundles, was vice president of the Mme. C. J. Walker Mfg. Co. while I was growing up. And my father, S. Henry Bundles, was president of another hair care products manufacturing company, Summit Laboratories, for nearly 20 years.

So the joys and dilemmas surrounding hair are not new to me. And while it might seem a contradiction to some to compare Madam Walker--a woman known for straightening hair--with Pamela Ferrell--a woman known for cultivating appreciation of natural hair--the parallels are striking.

In Pamela I see the tenacity and perseverance of Madam Walker, the entrepreneurial temperament and the polished professionalism. When Pamela takes on the beauty culture establishment, I see the warrior spirit that Madam Walker displayed in her support of the NAACP's anti-lynching movement. When Pamela and Taalib-Din fight for the rights of sisters who have exchanged welfare checks for checks from their braiding salon clients, I see the kind of empowerment Madam Walker envisioned when she created jobs for thousands of former sharecroppers and maids.

In 1919 Madam Walker told a reporter that her objective was not so much to straighten hair as to "have my people take a greater pride in their personal appearance and to give their hair proper attention...I dare say that in the next ten years it will be a rare thing to see a kinky head of hair and it will not be straight either." Although she was off by a few decades in her prediction and didn't fully anticipate the acceptance of locks and twists, perhaps Madam Walker was thinking of someone like Pamela Ferrell who could meld the American and African parts of our history to enhance our natural beauty.

In these pages Pamela bestows the gift of a fresh way of seeing, the gift of what she calls "freedom hair"--hair that is not a source of shame, hair that is not contorted into "unreal beauty standards." She reminds us that beauty begins within, then guides us through a self-love journey toward the realization that healthy hair--whether coily, kinky, straight, curly, nappy, crinkly or locked--is good hair.

Treat yourself to the restorative potion of Pamela's words so that when you touch your hair you will love what you feel.

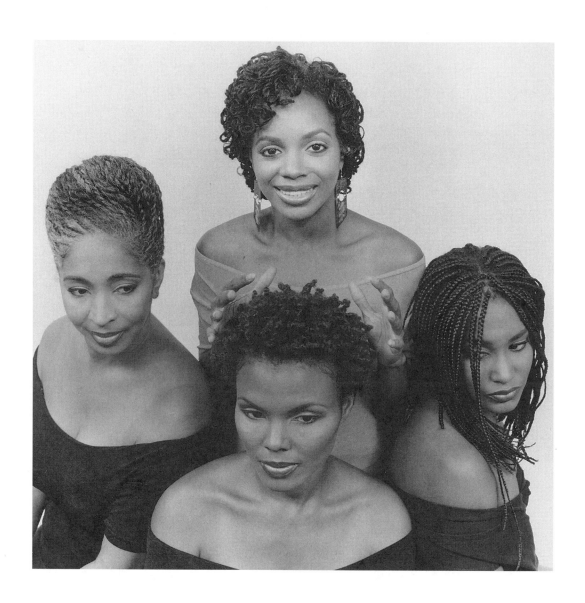

INTRODUCTION

This book is especially for black women who are committed to natural hair care, and for those who need to be. It is also an important read for men and for people of other ethnic origins, because feelings about hair are not only personal but, in many ways, reflective of the larger society's values. Those values have been horribly skewed and misdirected to the detriment of black women and their hair since the institution of slavery in the Americas.

Let's take a little test to show what I mean. In the total privacy of your heart, answer the following questions:

• Would you prefer to have been born with hair that's naturally wavy and silky or naturally tight-curled and wooly?

• When you hear the word "wooly" associated with hair, do you think of "hard and hard to comb" or "soft as lamb's wool" hair?

• Have you ever agreed with the adjectives "good" to describe hair that is naturally straight or loose-curled and "bad" for hair that is naturally tight-curled, kinky and nappy?

• Do the words "kinky" and "nappy" describe the kind of hair you find desirable?

• Are you embarrassed by the texture of your hair in its most natural state?

• Do you chemically straighten your hair regularly, to the point of damaging it, to achieve a non-nappy texture?

• Is "beautiful" a word you use to describe your hair in its natural state?

• What's your reaction to women who wear their hair naturally long and nappy?

• Have you accepted a standard of beauty that is incompatible with your natural attributes?

After you read this book, you'll understand why you answered those questions the way you did. You'll be able to put "hair" in its historical context, see the insidious racism that permeates much of the hair-care industry, and understand the connection between hair and health. Your answers may well change if you take the test a second time. Above all, "Let's Talk Hair" offers you the tools necessary for maintaining a healthy head of beautiful, desirable, natural hair -- tools I've shaped and fine-tuned during many years in the hair-care business.

Ready? Let's turn to Chapter One for a trip back in time, to a history that we will never let repeat itself.

Not all
black women
felt the need to
straighten their
hair.

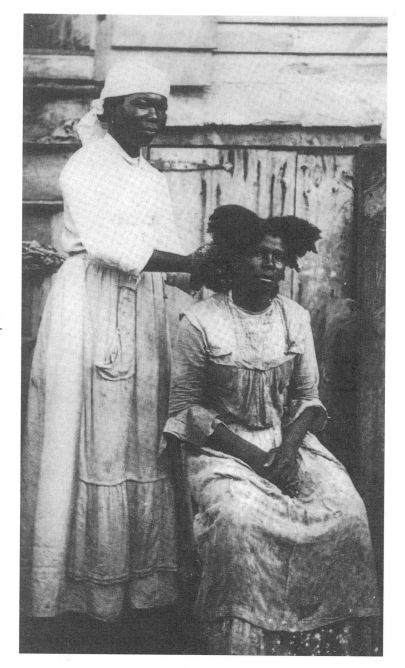

Plaiting hair 1900ca
Photographer unknown

The Battle
1
Of The Naps

Raped of her beauty

History has a way of repeating itself, especially if the bad is not challenged and the good not embraced. From the time the black woman set foot in America through today she has grappled with the troublesome issue of how to care for her hair and what styles are acceptable.

The African slave woman robbed and raped of her true sense of identity suffered the pain of being taken against her will from her homeland, sold from her family, treated as subhuman, and forced to abandon her name, dignity, and beauty. In the most de-humanizing conditions, survival became the order of life for the American black woman in slavery. She had to neglect her health and personal care under living conditions that lacked even the barest necessities and certainly not grooming utensils for curly, kinky hair.

The system of slavery socialized black people to feel inferior and fostered the beginnings of the negativism Africans in America came to face and, often, to adopt. African-American people were not born disliking themselves and their hair; rather, they learned this from the cruel circumstances they confronted as Africans in European-dominated worlds.

For these and other reasons, many African slave women learned to hate the color of their skin and the texture of their hair. These slave women and their descendants eventually saw themselves as untouched by beauty.

Black people also were victimized by the sexual exploitation of slave women by white slave masters that led to the "rainbow" of colors and hair textures in the race. As a matter of survival, fair skinned "colored people" with straight hair often chose to "pass" and be treated the same as white people; and lighter skinned slaves often were treated with less hostility by whites. However, the larger society typically looked down on dark complexioned people with curly, woolly hair.

As quiet as the black communities tried to keep it, they too learned to be prejudiced about skin color, and the quality and curliness of their own hair. Hair with less curl came to be called "good hair," while tight-curled hair was called "bad." Black people learned through fear to hate the hair God blessed them with and to hide, ridicule, and wage vehement warfare against its natural kink. Unfortunately, it has become commonplace to oppress the black woman's natural hair and innate beauty.

In the mid 1800s the black woman's hair was virtually outlawed in New Orleans when a city ordinance required all black female residents to wear a kerchief or tignon, over their heads.[1] Black women were required to put a scarf over their "coily" hair texture while out in public.

The African woman skilled in head wrapping made the best of ill circumstances and dressed her head with the simplest of rags. However, underneath she often neglected her hair. Poor hair care and limited grooming options caused serious hair and scalp problems. Historically, "Negro" women suffered from unhealthy hair, bald spots, and other scalp disorders because of the lack of time for grooming and the absence of beauty solutions designed to enhance the natural curl in their hair.

In the early 1900s, Madam C.J. Walker came to the black woman's rescue as one of the greatest beauty and hair care renegades of that time. She formulated hair cosmetics especially for the black woman's hair needs and encouraged these women to take pride in themselves. Her approach to hair care was wholistic, promoting the "healing effect" of such products as Wonderful Hair Grower and Vegetable Shampoo. Evidently, Madam Walker was compassionate about uplifting the black woman's image of herself; her advertisements never once denigrated black women's beauty. However, Madam Walker is mistakenly remembered for inventing the pressing comb, and portrayed as encouraging black women to alter their hair to resemble the European woman; and that's simply not true.

During Madam Walkers day, people debated whether black women should alter the appearance of their natural hair texture. A pioneer, Madam C.J. Walker insisted that her Walker Beauty System was not intended as a hair "straightener," but rather as part of a grooming method to heal and condition the scalp, to promote hair growth, and to make the hair easier to comb once it grew back. She was quoted in the Indianapolis

Recorder in 1919: *"Right here let me correct the erroneous impression held by some that I claim to straighten the hair,"* she told a reporter. *"I want the great masses of my people to take a greater pride in their personal appearance and to give their hair proper attention."* [2]

Madam Walker considered her hot combing method to be more natural and an improvement over previous practices using a device called the "hair puller," popularized by her competitor, Annie Malone, that flattened the hair strands straight. The "flat iron," as we know it today, is used by beauticians to straighten black women's already chemically straightened hair beyond recognition.

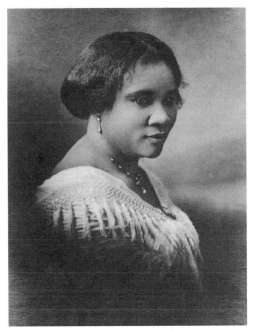

Madam C.J. Walker 1910
Photo courtesy, The Walker Collection of Alelia Bundles

Unfortunately, the "battle of the naps" gained momentum as straightened hair became the popular style for the black woman. Whether to please her oppressor, to feel more beautiful, or to gain power in a society that offered little opportunity for the black woman to be noticed, she soon realized that straightening her hair was less offensive than wearing her nappy tresses. The Negro hair dresser and white-owned companies with products like "Kinkilla" perpetuated the negative idea of "fixing" the black woman's natural hair. From this, the "cosmetic conspiracy" had its debut.

Cosmetic companies took advantage of the fragile, insecure black woman. They understood that she was in a constant struggle to find the time, money and where-with-all to care for her hair. Knowing she took little pride in her natural hair, it was not difficult to appeal to her need to "correct" and alter its "ugliness." This philosophy still maintains a stronghold on black American women today. Because of this, all beauty regimens for black women's hair were designed with the intent of hiding or "correcting" its nappy, curly condition.

Pomade and the straightening comb became a dynamic duo in the hands of a beautician whose job was to eliminate the natural nap of the black woman's hair at any cost. She waged valiant warfare against her arch enemies, water and perspiration, which invariably caused the straightened hair to revert to its natural, nappy state. For this reason, many black women disdained sports, exercise (especially swimming) lest they "sweat out" their straightened hair and cause it to "go back." Needless to say, this endless, futile war with nature fattened the pockets of the black beautician and continues to encourage black women to seek a false identity.

Madam Walker intended her pressing comb invention to make the black woman's hair easier to comb, not to make the hair duplicate Caucasian hair texture. But over time, in the hands of the beautician, it became the tool to eliminate nap and create "silky hair." Still this was not enough; this was too temporary.

After a long search for a permanent solution to the problem of temporary straight hair, in the1940s women were offered the permanent lye-based chemical relaxer. Once again the cosmetics industry profited richly. Today a multi-billion dollar industry offers hair relaxers, perms, and even kiddie perms for today's black children. It was not difficult to sell the idea of straightening the hair, because many black women had learned to hate their coily hair. The "perm" presented a great opportunity for the cosmetics industry to take advantage of black women and their quest for "good hair."

The products created to fix the black women's hair imply that somehow God made a mistake, and black people were born with "bad" hair; therefore, they need to buy something or pay somebody to help them achieve a "good" hair texture.

It is important to note that not all black women felt the need to straighten their natural hair, even as the trend leaned toward rebuking naps. Some were content with grooming and styling the hair naturally, and never adopted the larger culture's standard of beauty.

Cosmetology restrictions

Unfortunately, Eurocentric institutions, cosmetic manufacturers and mis-educated "Negroes" who push the notion that black women should straighten out the natural, coily texture of their hair and seek the all-American (white) beauty ideal, still lead the charge of the cosmetology industry. Today, the cosmetology trade has built an institution on promoting one standard of beauty and qualifying hair texture.

On June 7, 1938, Congress passed the cosmetology act for the District of Columbia that established the law to regulate the trade of cosmetology. Trade regulations disguised as ways to protect the consumer's health and safety were actually created to restrict entry into certain trades, including hair care. White cosmetology schools did not admit black students so black schools opened to accommodate them; however, the black salons and schools had to comply with regulations set by their white competitors. The beauty school curriculum and license exams were never relevant to safe hair care for African-Americans. For example, the cosmetology license exam, then and now, requires a model with straight hair. As recently as June 1995, I witnessed African-American cosmetology examiners say the reason a black student failed "skip waves" was because her black model's hair was not straight enough. They postured as if they were authorities on the black woman's hair, as they were firmly upholding a nationwide cosmetology exam that perpetuates the white woman's hair texture as the standard for proficient practice.

Cosmetology laws in other states mirror the District of Columbia 1938 cosmetology act. Many states have not changed or revised their outdated rules or exams. It is common knowledge that laws created to regulate did not include the Negro but could control their participation in the trade. As African Americans were busy with the civil rights struggle, fighting for the right to ride in the front of buses, patronize any restaurant, etc., our right to free enterprise, especially in the hair-care industry (even within our communities), was under attack and legislated away.

Cosmetology boards across the nation practice regulatory racism. I know of hair braiders from Texas, Ohio, Illinois, New Jersey, California, Pennsylvania, Florida, South and North, Carolina, Tennesse, Michigan, and others states who are harassed and threatened by cosmetology board members. They have gone so far as to show up at the hair braider's salon and verbally intimidate the braider to cease braiding until she obtains a cosmetology license that qualifies her to straighten the black woman's hair. Even though the 1930's outdated cosmetology laws were never intended to include African-American hair care or braiding, they claim to regulate braiding. The original intent of this law was not to care for all types of hair but, rather, to test the proficiency of straight hair styling. The text books written by white publishers in the 1930's, which are still used in cosmetology schools today, do not include African-American hair care. Even though African-American women Kathryn Wilson and Madam C.J. Walker published cosmetology textbooks in the 1920s, their books are seldom, if at all, found in black cosmetology schools. Instead the standard textbook used in cosmetology schools are straight hair-oriented, while curly, kinky hair texture is denigrated. Kinky hair texture is professionally referred to as "overcurly," as if the curl is too much. One textbook author writes "there is little doubt that the over-curly hair is a special form of terminal hair. Experts can explain little about its origin but suggest it is caused by a difference in the papilla and germinal matrix in the follicles of the people concerned. Over-curly hair is difficult to handle and comb." [3] However, this same textbook speaks on the positive "natural" features and causes of straight and wavy hair. Cosmetologists learn from textbooks that have a blatant disregard for curly, kinky hair. Class instructions, even in black cosmetology schools, teach European hair styles, such as finger waves and pin curls which are required training for cosmetology examination, although the techniques could not be done on the black woman's natural hair texture.

In May 1982 I unknowingly challenged the State of Maryland Cosmetology Board by bringing an African American female model with natural hair for my state board haircut. The examiner failed me because she did not know how to check the hair cut on curly textured hair. After I challenged the requirement of straight textured hair, the Maryland State Board of cosmetology did something that has never been done in the history of cosmetology state board exams: they provided me with a model, a Caucasian model with straight hair, in order for me to re-do my state board exam hair cut or face a discrimination lawsuit. I passed the exam.

For years, the majority of black hair dressers complied with cosmetology regulations that exclude hair braiding. They conformed and knowingly participated in an industry that had no concern for natural hair care or the African American aesthetic. Hair braiders who felt excluded from this industry offered hair care that was strikingly different, rather than participate in corrective cosmetology. To chemically straighten the black woman's hair was against American hair braider's principles and not an option to healthy hair care.

To gain control or thwart the growth of the braiding business, boards of cosmetology across the United States attempted to regulate the practice of hair braiding even though they knew nothing about it and would have preferred to outlaw it. In 1980 Cornrows & Co., the premier hair braiding salon, launched what became an 11-year challenge to the District of Columbia's 1938 regulation that excluded hair braiding. After scores of correspondence, four attorneys, three introductions of proposed legislation, 14 appearances before the Board of Cosmetology, four council hearings, two fines, one cease and desist order, four department investigations, one civil adjudication court procedure and appeal, two mayoral administrations and one federal lawsuit, the District government finally changed the law to define a specialty hair braider's license. On January 3, 1993, Mayor Sharon Pratt Kelly signed a new law that included hair braiding as "specialty cosmetology." This historical change in the law recognizes hair braiding salons, hair braiding schools, instructors and natural hair care as a specialized discipline of beauty care, creating a standard for the growing hair braiding and natural hair care industry.

Freedom hair

In the mid 1960s, the militant black power movement and re-birth of black pride created an environment for a new black aesthetic. A hair style called the Afro was born in black American communities. Black people from coast to coast learned to enjoy the splendid luxury of their natural hair. In fact, even white people began to ask their beauticians for a permanent that would add nap and kink to their hair. Pride, self respect and embracing black heritage began to overturn centuries of shame and fear. Black people discovered their identity and expressed it in a new-found liberation with their natural hair. Straightening the "Afro" hair was no longer in vogue. Even Jewish people who were chastised for their kinky hair texture found liberation during this "self-pride" movement. They, too, could throw away the "Get it straight" hair product and appreciate the natural curl in their hair.

Black women and men felt pride in themselves, in spite of the "old school" Negroes who would disown their own brothers, sisters, sons, daughters and anyone who chose to wear the "Afro." For the first time, black people were able to pocket the money that had been financing the "corrective" beauty culture. At the same time, however, black cosmetologists and cosmetics companies suffered financial losses because the Afro hair style required little or no professional maintenance nor straightening products. So they pushed products designed to change the natural texture and helped advance the notion that the Afro was merely a fad hair style. Thirty years later, young kids who did not live in the "black power" era are wearing the cornrows and the Afro with pride. When I hear my 8-year-old nephew proudly speak of growing his "bush" as if this is a new style, I feel some sense of comfort. I realize, though, that unless he appreciates the true beauty of his hair and its relationship to his identity, he will fall victim to viewing his natural hair as a fad. If he learns to appreciate his natural hair, it will not just become a style with no real significance, nor an in-between style before the Geri-curl fad recycles.

Even though the mid to late 1960s "Black is Beautiful" movement was short lived, the memory gave men and women a period of pride and freedom in styling their hair. The "I'm black and I'm proud" era cultivated a new generation of proud parents. It was one of the most empowering for black hair care, but it fell prey to the industry. The 1970s chemical hair care era replaced black pride with the "conservative" straightened hair look. Many black women became convinced once more that they "needed to look more white and less black." The 1980s began the period of blatant hair style restrictions and discrimination. In cities across America, natural and braided styles were vehemently opposed by an economy that had made billions of dollars promoting a mentality among black people that their natural hair is inappropriate, unprofessional and ugly. This was especially echoed in educational institutions and in the workplace. Young women leaving African-American college campuses on their professional exodus are forewarned by career counselors and job recruiters to remove their braids, straighten their natural hair and hide their African-American identity. These counselors teach the graduates that intelligence and good character are not as important as conforming to white America's beauty ideals. Even though this message may solve the immediate concern of getting hired, the long-term effect again forces black women to be unnatural. Hair texture becomes the qualifying factor for success or failure. The most important message the campus recruiters can impart to young women is the importance of good character, a clean neat and healthy appearance, and job skills. To pass on their fears is counter-productive for developing high self-esteem. Job recruiters may be trying to shelter young job seekers from the harsh realities of corporate America, and some of these recruiters may themselves be responsible for enforcing the anti-braid, anti-black corporate policies.

Within major corporations and government offices, black supervisors often are called upon to enforce anti-braid, European inspired dress code policies. They bring the threat that you will lose your job or lose the opportunity to gain advancement within the job if you wear a hair style that is non-European.

In 1978 while in college, I lost my part-time job as a fabric store clerk after being warned by my black supervisor on behalf of the stores owner to remove my braids. Even though I knew it was wrong, I believed that within time things would change so that black women would not be subjected to hair style discrimination and threats of losing their jobs. To my disappointment, nine years later 1987, I received a telephone call at my hair braiding salon from Cheryl Tatum who was fired from her job at the Hyatt Hotel in Crystal City, VA. because she choose to wear a braided hair style. This was a sign for me that this problem would not go away with time and that black women could not sit back and participate in this kind of racism.

In 1992 I received another telephone call from another hotel employee, Pam Mitchell, who was angry because she was threatened for wearing a braid style. Management at the Washington, DC JW Marriott Hotel gave her a Christmas eve ultimatum, "Remove your braid style or lose your job." The matter was settled and Pam Mitchell returned to her work with her braided hair style, a $55,000. settlement and a raise.

The threat of a law suit, which would expose unwarranted racism, garnered results. Cornrows & Co. with the help of Attorney Eric Steele filed class action suits against major hotels and corporations across the country. Through this effort black women discovered that they already have the rights they sought and only needed to exercise them. In the 1990s, black women continue to face the dilemma of making a choice to forgo their dignity and rights in order to keep a job and feed their families.

The District of Columbia's Police Department and the Smithsonian Institute's security force also was challenged for their anti-braid policy, which changed as a result of media exposure. Black women insisted that dress and hair codes must reflect the multi-ethnic workplace. Natural curly hair is quite different from Caucasian straight hair, so hair style regulations should be general enough for anyone to realistically meet (such as, above the collar, neat, clean and fits easily under head gear).

A demonstration was given before the United States Navy board of dress regulations that showed a braided hair style was more practical for African-American female officers who are ship-bound for an extended time. In November 1994 we celebrated another victory, the US Navy anti-braid policy was abolished. Black female officers are wearing braids in the United States Navy, the last US military agency to change its dress code to recognize braid styles.

In 1994, Cornrows & Co. filed another class action suit against American Airlines for its anti-braid policy. Flight attendant Barbara Cooper called our salon, hurt by what she termed a "double blow." Her black female supervisor, whom she admired, gave her the ultimatum to unbraid her hair or lose her job. Racism has many perpetrators but the same victim, the African American.

The battle of the naps had taken a new direction. Black women were no longer willing to sit back in fear and witness a blatant disregard for their right to wear natural hair styles. Word had gotten out that the Cornrows & Co. salon was willing to support women emotionally and legally if they were threatened with losing their jobs because of their braid styles. The salon was no longer just a place of beautification; it had become a refuge where women could gain support in their fight for "freedom hair."

I have cited a few cases to show that the right to wear African-inspired hair styles will continue to be challenged by anyone who feels threatened, black or white. A natural hair style or stylist is an affront to the hair care industry, with its anti-braid policies, hair gels, glues, relaxers, and spritzers ready to enforce every strand of hair and prevent black women from loving their natural curly kinky hair. Whether this kind of display is based on greed or is racially motivated is not the issue. My deepest concern is the damage this kind of racism, hype and frenzy over straight hair texture has done to the black female's self esteem and hair follicles.

Define your own beauty standard

No matter how you wear your hair, there will always be someone to disapprove, scrutinize, or admire it. Often family, friends, companions, co-workers, employers and people who don't even know you will comment. They judge your beauty or lack of it continuously. Some women unfortunately fashion their beauty to please others, while other women do not allow society to dictate what is beautiful for them. They have made a conscious decision to not get caught up in the self-defeating cycle of trying to please others. They realize the person to please is themselves. Every woman does not possess an eye for beauty, and may make a mistake that causes her to look less attractive; however, this does not give someone else the right to make her feel ugly. Remember this: any comments from others about your choice of style should be thoughtful and instructive, not judgmental.

The best teachers for sharing beauty ideas and suggestions are loving, knowing females who have the same attributes and purpose for beauty as you. Such a woman will help you ponder questions like, "What makes me feel unquestionably beautiful?" "What feels good to me and is good for my health?" "How do I see myself?" Only you can answer these questions, to ultimately choose the best self-image. Self identity is realized when women dismiss harsh and unrealistic beauty standards engendered by a society of disrespectful audiences.

Fashion and beauty ideals are not always created by the people who are to uphold them. Men who design skin-tight dresses and crotch suffocating pants would never wear these things for the sake of beauty. But many women feel they must suffer dis-comfort to be part of the "attractive and alluring" beauty standard. Too many black women are caught up in the all American standard of beauty, a standard that even most white women cannot uphold, and should not have to either. Each woman has her own innate loveliness, and that should be the standard by which she measures herself. Trying to be an all American beauty can leave the most attractive woman feeling psychologically defeated and untouched by beauty. I often see women strug-gling physically, emotionally, and financially to fashion their physical attributes to meet an impossible criteria.

Men are rarely the subject of beauty and do not concern themselves with the color and texture of their hair, or what products will make it alluring and attractive. They are simply consumers of our beauty, not understanding what is physically, emotionally and spiritually involved in enhancing it. They sit back and enjoy the Miss America, Miss Universe and Miss whoever exudes the most beauty, and many expect all women to measure up. Even businessmen see great financial benefit in portraying the female to be attractive, sexually appealing, with luxurious hair. They use her image to sell prod-ucts and the illusion that the product will make anyone as beautiful. They envision what they like in a woman and appeal to the female's desire to feel beautiful and admired. Unfortunately they do not care about the psychological impact unreal beauty standards have on the female and male psyches. Many cosmetic and hair product companies are owned by men, and the marketing and advertising decisions are seldom made by women. Beauty campaigns are organized by the businessmen who stand to gain the most by creating an impossible beauty criteria, such as the one-dimensional beauty ideal that women believe they can buy. I once talked with a mar-keting executive of a manufacturing company for synthetic fiber for wigs and hair extensions; he told me he thought black women wore wigs because they cannot grow hair, and since sales had gone down he wanted to know what was wrong and how could he plan a marketing program to sell the black woman more wigs and extensions. It struck me that men hold their board meetings to create images and standards of beauty without considering the woman's point of view and her realities. Their goal is to sell the illusion of beauty and to increase their financial bottom line.

No more hair struggles

Historically, African and Native American women were groomed by caring females who understood it was the woman's place to care for and beautify other women. There were rites of passage where older, knowledgeable women taught young women the secrets of personal care. This was the mystique of the female beauty;

more than just cosmetic embellishments, these knowing women were responsible for promoting the female's mental, physical and spiritual well-being. A complete approach to beauty.

Unfortunately, this tradition suffered when the African woman came to America in slavery. Her priorities did not allow her to concentrate on initiation rites into womanhood. Her well-being and complete happiness were put on the back burner while she tended to everyone else's needs. She accepted her thankless role of being all to everybody. From her beginning in America, the black female was taught not to complain nor question the things that brought her the most discomfort.

Black women have struggled for so long with every element of their existence in America that the pain and suffering over their beauty is a natural consequence. The female child felt the brunt of these frustrations early on from the mother who felt overburdened and powerless. She unknowingly passed the hardship on to her young daughter. Included among these frustrations is the American woman's "struggle of hair and beauty," a sort of initiation. The biggest part of the struggle is the great effort to make our hair opposite to its natural attributes. These are the lessons the young black female learns today, mis-guided and self destructive to her God given beauty.

The womanhood stories about getting your hair pressed, the pulling, the tugging, the good hair-bad hair, the light skin-dark skin, anti-African and pro-European aesthetic are all the things we spend so much time cultivating. It's no wonder the black woman struggles with her hair and self image. Many do not even know it, and subconsciously accept as a natural misfortune being born with the kind of hair that is hard to comb, shrinks in the rain, isn't silky, your man can't run his fingers through, and countless other reasons to justify battling with the glorious head of hair God has blessed you with. I know God makes no mistakes, and the black woman's hair texture is not one. The struggle with hair is only her reality if she accepts it. Attempting to change what you have little control over is a no-win battle. As long as any woman dislikes her natural hair, and attempts to make it into an opposing texture, that becomes her battle. With the many grooming tips and styles designed for natural hair, any black woman can now be selective about not altering her hair. In the process, she may realize that true beauty is within her and not in the products or hair extensions she can buy. The pressure of meeting unreal beauty standards will then go away, as will the denial of her follicle condition. Once you decide not to fight your natural hair you will feel liberated as if you lifted a self-imposed burden off yourself.

Turn the page to start your journey within and end all battles with your hair.......

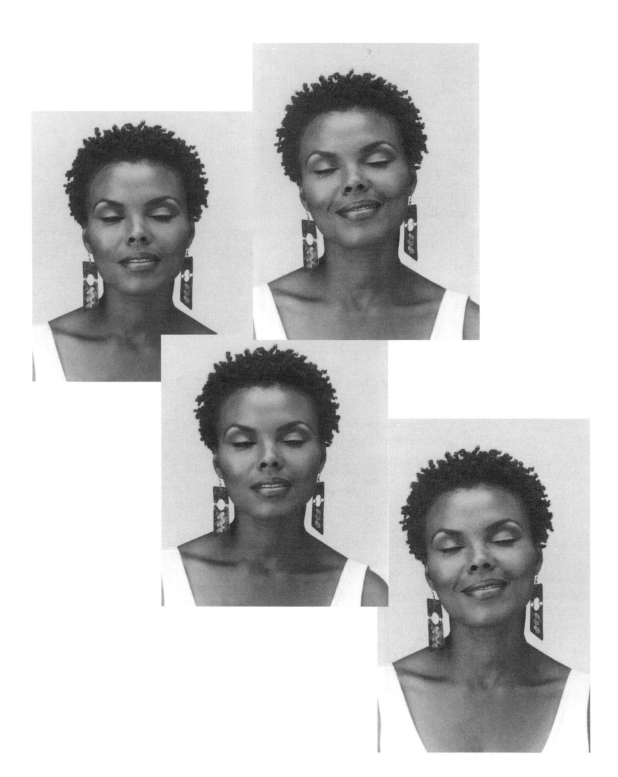

The Journey 2 Within Yourself

Your inside beauty

As a natural hair care advocate, I encourage women to adore, respect and appreciate their God-given loveliness and understand that good hair and beauty start within. I am a guide, to share my expertise and support during the quest to discover inner beauty.

My biggest challenge is realizing I cannot make anyone change their self image or behavior. I can help a woman appreciate her beauty if she wants to herself. Wellness and healthy hair care are two things she must desire. I can provide the information, style ideas, a place of natural care and beauty regimen, but each woman is responsible for using it. That is the reason I am always grateful for clients who are motivated and sincere in participating in their health and beauty care.

There is nothing more marvelous and fascinating than the evolving female. If she is nurtured and given the right circumstances her growth can be a joyful experience. Even the mature woman who may feel that with age her beauty diminishes, if she is given the opportunity to develop in a positive enriching environment her inside beauty only gets better with age. Wisdom, maturity and confidence are just a few of the attributes that give her a secure sense of inside beauty that forms from the ongoing experiences and the many people who cross her life path. These things will shape the way we understand and feel about ourselves, both good and bad. Even though there is a born instinct to love oneself, a rude external environment and crude people can change that natural tendency.

Years of being in the hair and beauty industry have shown me the deep down ugly side of people. I witness first hand the behavior of fragile and desperate women who have learned to dislike themselves, hate their hair texture, and do harmful things to change it -- actions that epitomize self hate.

One of the first things I try to cultivate in my female client is a positive mental outlook about herself and life in general. This is paramount for good health and happiness. We can find so many things to complain about, from soft hair to nappy edges, when we should be thankful for simply having hair. As we entertain these negative thoughts our mind wastes time and energy, not realizing if we change the way we think we can change the way we feel.

The mind is one of the greatest healing agents. With it we can develop the ability to visualize complete happiness, good health and beauty. For example, if you see yourself as being ugly, overworked and poor, you will continue to live that existence as long as you visualize and apply it. If you truly believe you are ugly, the "I hate myself" attitude will begin to manifest that idea into action, and that becomes a fulfilling goal. The more you tell yourself this, the more it becomes your reality. No one can love you better than you, nor hate you worse than yourself. In fact, it is perfectly healthy and okay to love yourself, and if you have not been doing this, it is time to begin now.

A different, more loving outlook naturally creates a loving self, and a healthy experience. It is helpful to begin to re-examine the way you feel about yourself and ask-- Where did I get my beauty ideals? What influenced my deep self hate? Why am I so critical and negative about my hair? What makes me feel beautiful? These are a few of the questions you will answer to develop your beauty within. Once you begin to view yourself positively, you can accept and believe that passing stranger who gives you a sincere compliment about your beauty. The inner beauty of your soul will shine through so others may see.

When I talk about inner beauty it is the difference between a woman who walks into a room full of people and is noticed for her fantastic hair style or the woman who walks in and is remembered because of her radiance and assured presence, where everything about her is beautiful. We have all seen this type of beautiful woman and remember the little things as well as the entire spirit. The love she exudes from within touches many people who are searching for inner peace and beauty.

The outside influence

As a topic of discussion, the black woman's hair opens a view to African-American culture and family. Few other subjects will cause black people to unveil their feelings and relate deeply personal experiences. Discussions about hair may start with childhood stories, job standards, bad hair days, or the pretty hair style seen on someone else. In the salon I can start talking with one or two persons, others will overhear the "hair conversation" and soon there will be a high-spirited gathering of women pouring out personal stories, anecdotes, and much laughter.

In much of the black community (as perhaps in American society as a whole), hair is viewed as the ultimate in a woman's beauty. If it is long and wavy, the woman is considered beautiful with "good hair." She may also be disliked because of her "good hair" texture. And a dark skinned woman with long hair is still looked at as if this is abnormal. An example is the comment a dark-skinned female with long, beautiful hair is subjected to: "She has pretty hair to be so dark," as if dark skin and long hair do not go together.

By the age of 8, black girls learn the importance of hair and what type and quality are more desirable. On my travels throughout the United States I have found in the black communities people will speak freely about hair. As different as the geographic lifestyles may be, the subject of hair is always an intricate part of the socialization of the community. You can tell a lot about that community based on how hair is valued or de-valued.

As I listen to the variety of hair tales, I am able to gather a common consensus about how that black community views the female's beauty and her hair. Beauty is always about the female. You will seldom hear in-depth discussions about a man's beauty, and if so his manhood comes into question. Men are not necessarily the source of beauty. They are consumers of it because they judge it, desire it and look for it. The young woman learns, too, that she is always on display and a subject of debate and that her happiness in life could be contingent on her meeting these beauty standards. In reality, every woman has something attractive about her; no matter how far her beauty features are from the desired norm, there will always be a man who will adore her for that special something.

As women gather and continuously discuss the subject of hair, I am able to hear the patterns of influence. Her community, the church, workplace, home life and parent's beauty ideals all affect how the female views her hair. I guide my clients to look back into their childhood and recollect the experiences they had. This is a way of getting a woman to open up and talk about experiences that are dormant within her psyche, and inadvertently direct her actions today.

Many women who talk about their childhood hair experiences with laughter are able to analyze those experiences with less stress and pressure. Laughter is one route to healing. Many of the stories are quite funny and pitiful at the same time. These stories are a keyhole into American culture as it relates to hair and beauty, candid stories that tell of the self hatred perpetuated in the African-American community and family and a crucial and ongoing part of the female upbringing. If you want people to open up and talk about their family, ask them about getting their hair "done."

The first part of the "journey within" is to gather past information about your hair experiences. Work up to now and take inventory of where you are today and how you feel about yourself. *Are you dis-satisfied with your hair?*
Do you feel overwhelmed when trying to care for your hair?
Is it frustrating, impossible, depressing, and difficult to style?
Do you worry how other people view your hair?
Have you been feeling as if something is not right about your hair?

If you have answered yes to any of the questions, you can evaluate your negative feelings and find solutions for enjoyable hair care that is less stressful. Let's read on.... Your childhood experiences (good or bad) are a start for self examination. You are not alone in this need for hair freedom and self discovery. A change is taking place among masses of black women who are tired of fighting their hair, disliking themselves, using caustic cosmetics and desiring styles that are not designed for their hair.

The African-American woman is awakening to the reality that she can experiment and enjoy her own natural loveliness. Through this she will accept and get to know her own hairs beauty. This is not to say that other races of people accept themselves more. Other races of women dislike their hair, skin color, and physical attributes too.

My focus is simply on healthy hair care for the African-American woman, and how to inspire her away from the materialistic preoccupations, back to a spiritual alignment of nurturing and caring for herself.

When is the last time you took a journey within? Quietly sat and prayed, meditated and listened to your deep thoughts? Answered the questions only you know the answers to? Complimented and adored yourself? Directed your attention from your physical body to your spiritual and mental self, by not only engaging in the tangible things you can see and touch, but the intangible things such as emotions, feeling, spirituality and intuition.

Dealing with the deep inside sensations like feeling ugly, not feeling noticed because your hair is too short and other emotional experiences can leave deep scars and hidden anxiety. As a way to not self examine, we construct inside walls of defense and protection from revisiting painful experiences. The unhappy experiences we dismiss as incidental. We set up false facades that give the impression that we are so together and have not had any problems in our lives. This is reason enough to journey inward and start chipping away at the barriers that restrain you from confronting your true self. Only you can make your inward journey.

If you tune into yourself and listen to your instincts, you will find that your intuition is very accurate. Women have learned to take instinctive knowing for granted and ignore it as if it is not what we expect. Our internal self is very much in touch with the external forces. We are like body sponges and we pick up stuff we don't realize we can absorb. We consume all the silly beauty myths, fears, society's hang-ups and negative conditioning from external forces that continually leave false impressions.

We will accumulate a lot of inner baggage that can impede our growth and development unless we are aware and listen to our intuition. Inner burdens can cause us to feel weighted down and too tired to confront them. This can make the inward journey at first difficult or impossible for some women. Some of us will travel lightly while others will need to lighten the load. This is like taking a flight where the cargo is too much. One of two things will happen; either the plane cannot take off or if it does take off it will become imbalanced and have to make a crash landing. We all know it is a lot more difficult to look for clues from a wreckage than to take precautionary measures before taking off.

As with any other journey it helps to be prepared, know where you are coming from and your destination. This enables you to be alert and open to the many signs that can make your personal journey within successful. If the unexpected should happen in the process it is by divine direction and there is a lesson to gain from it. There may be people and situations in life that we must learn from; even the ones that appear as bad experiences may bring the most valuable lessons to our life. Let us prepare for the journey by back tracking into childhood. What kind of parents did you have? How did family members react to your physical beauty? When you were a small child, did your family marvel and make a fuss over your looks or were you the ugly duckling? These simple questions will give you an idea of your early messages.

A place for healing

My salon has been more than a place for getting a beautiful hair style; it has become a place for healing. Historically, it has been uncommon for African-American women to go to a psychologist, psychiatrist, or other therapist -- a "shrink" as it's commonly referred to. People fear being considered "crazy" rather than having some stressing issues to talk about and work on. Consequently, the hair stylist often becomes the therapist and psychoanalyst to her clients. She also is a confidant, sister, and friend. A woman may tell her braider, hair stylist private matters that she may not express to anyone else.

On any given day at my salon, which has open space with no distractions like television and toxic fumes from chemicals, women will talk in the traditional way. The space is reminiscent of "women's circles" where women can freely talk about female "secrets" and girl things. Some women cannot find this camaraderie anywhere else. Although many women were blessed to have a family of women or an extended family to experience regular female gatherings, this era of concentration on material gain leaves little time to sit down and chat. The closest to this is the occasional bridal or baby shower where females can talk about "women's stuff", free of the male presence.

The African and Native American tradition nurtured the female gender with initiations, rites of passage and women's groupings. The wise and knowing elder women always guided the young females. For women who seldom have the opportunity to engage in positive relationships with other women, the hair salon can fill this void. The natural hair care salon is a place, additionally, where women can exchange thoughts and be consoled by someone they believe to have answers to long unaddressed questions.

At the salon, a woman will get a temporary external boost from a beautiful hair style and lasting internal work on the quest to achieve self love. She develops an intimate and trusting relationship with the natural care stylist who handles her head, the crown and highest part of the body. Not all braiders and natural stylists have the gift to heal and make their clients feel whole, probably because that is not their intention. This kind of relationship and offering can take years to establish and develop. It requires intuitive instincts.

Clients who come to me talk about personal issues, how they feel about themselves (good and bad), and comment about their family and friends. They feel safe enough to talk about relationships with parents and/or male companions. Some clients have been in tears, so relieved to get feelings out in the open. In these impromptu sessions, I work to help my female client appreciate and love herself and to look at her situation differently, to stop blaming herself and feeling she has the world on her shoulders. It is fundamental for her to let go of negative thoughts and emotions, so that she will value herself and take care of her own happiness as she attempts to do for others. One of the issues that regularly emerges during the "personal salon session" is how the woman's close friends and family confuse her opinion of herself and her hair.

I always try to start with family and childhood memories. Inevitably things that were troubling in childhood carry on into adult relationships and personal perceptions. I learned that a young girl who is raised solely by a father or male is likely to have a different outlook and perspective about herself than the female reared by a woman. The female who does not have a father or loving male presence in her life has different challenges in becoming secure about her beauty.

Parents play perhaps the most important role in how we learn to see ourselves. They can nurture us into secure, self-loving beings, or push us toward insecurity, insanity, and unhappiness -- often without intending to do it. Each client's childhood story and salon sessions are individualized and geared to their one-of-a kind needs. You may not see yourself in any of the following types. Your childhood experience may be all together different, but we can all learn from each other.

The motherless female

The relationship between the client and female natural hair care stylist often goes well beyond hair care. The stylist may be a substitute mother in the motherless female's life, a mother only in the sense that she can offer female love and support to someone who had too little of it in her life. All females need mother relationships -- support, guidance, caring and love from wise, knowing women.

A young girl needs a mother role model to teach her the basics of female grooming and tell the young female how beautiful she is. Being viewed as beautiful is essential in nurturing good self esteem and teaching self-love and personal value. It enables girls to create healthy relationships with other women so that they do not have to feel competitive, insecure or less beautiful. A mother's presence can teach the female side of love along with personal hygiene, grooming and hair care.

Fathers who are raising daughters need the support of extended family (sisters, aunts, neighbors) in raising a female child. It is challenging for a woman to rear a male child alone; it can be equally problematic for a male to rear a female.

Some lessons can be learned best from another who has passed through the same developmental stages. A man may not be the best teacher for a woman about her body and childbirth. A woman may not be best suited to teach her son about manhood. This is not to say that all mothers can teach the female side of life, or all men the male side. There, too, is the unknowing parent who is like a child without the experience and knowledge to teach a child self love and development.

The unaffectionate mother

If your mom smothered you with hugs and kisses, consider yourself blessed. For some women this tender and attentive treatment all souls crave has been missing in their lives. The unloved female raised by a mother who did not know how to express her love or affection is at a loss for the most basic part of nurturing. Perhaps the mother, too, lacked this experience and ended up feeling helpless and indifferent, and her children suffer because of it.

Then there is the child who may have been tormented or verbally abused by her mother. Lacking an uplifting word or supportive embrace, she becomes fragile and may end up looking for love in all the wrong places, always expecting the worst since she has never known better. I have talked to many women who resent how their mothers treat them and fear confronting it as an adult.

Some young girls remember being reminded constantly about their "bad" hair and ugliness inherited from the "other side of the family." These are mean-spirited things to constantly tell a child. The adult female replays these negative memories that were often told to her by the person she admired, trusted and looked up to. When you lose trust in your mother it is difficult to trust yourself. To make matters even worse, some females were constantly reminded how inadequate their beauty is compared to other girls or even other siblings. A mother's lack of loving attention and ignorance may very well be the cause of her self-aversion. Once this behavior starts, it can continue for generations. A mistreated woman may treat her child the same way, or become so numb to this type of ill treatment that she continues to involve herself in unloving relationships, which she may think are normal. When was the last time your mother hugged or kissed you? When is the last time you hugged or kissed your child?

The fatherless female

"Daddy's little girl" may be the story book tale that some females never lived. There simply was not a dad in their life. And if the mother moved away from the extended family, she took uncles and grand-dads out of the little girl's life, too. Men show a female child the male side of affection and feelings. It has been my experience that male siblings and family members teach the many sides of love.

My brother and male cousins used to "crack on me" (make fun of) while we walked to church. They would talk about my skinny legs, big head and funny hairdo. The more it bothered me, the better their jokes got. I soon learned to laugh with them and realized they have a foolish way of expressing their love and telling you how pretty you really are. They, too, would fight any other male that made fun of me; only they had that right. It is a healthy reality check for the female to not internalize the immature male's silly jokes and to see them simply as one way of expressing love.

The male can help the female become more secure about her own likes and dislikes. One female client who never met her dad would get so bothered and defensive about how men looked at her; yet she would wear hairdos that were eye-catching, and voluptuous clothes that were snug and scanty. On the one hand she hated men for their "doggish ways," but on the other hand she yearned for their attention without understanding why she wanted it. Perhaps a father would have taught her that her beauty was not to be compromised, instilled confidence in her so that she would not suspect that a man has lewd motives whenever he gives her a sincere, respectful compliment.

Fathers can be so important to help the female feel secure and beautiful. The father who intimidates, who verbally abuses his female child, especially about her hair and her beauty, may as well be an absent father. If he is domineering and unnerving, his daughter will likely be insecure and untrusting with men.

The controlling parent

Guiding parents teach their children how to make decisions and develop into responsible adults. Then there are parents who want to make all the decisions and control every strand of their child's hair. I have witnessed parents who come to the salon with their daughters to consult about having the child's hair done. The parent selects the style and all the details about it. Sometimes the child may want something different but the parent is bent on choosing the hair style she wants the child to wear.

The parent will ask the child what color beads she would like, the child chooses red and then the parent says "no I think black is better." I realize that the parent is paying for the hair service, and feels she knows best; however, it is helpful to let a child feel some sense of involvement, especially since the child has to wear the hair style and feel good about herself. If a child never participates in a decision that involves her appearance, she will grow up not being able to make decisions for herself or resenting guidance and suggestions. Rebelling against adults may be her sense of independence. Then the controlling parent is left wondering why her child is out of control.

A child as young as 3 years old knows what hair style she likes and dislikes. She has a voice and knows how a style feels. If your child complains that cornrows are tight and she prefers loose braids, only she knows how her head feels. Of course as the parent you may set some boundaries, such as giving the child a dollar amount that you are willing to pay for the hair style, and perhaps explaining that the hair style must be suitable for her age. This at least gives the child something to work within rather than a hair style that you pay for and the child hates. How would you feel if someone made you wear a hair style you hated? Less control and more guidance can nurture a secure happy female.

Insecure lovers

An insecure woman will inevitably attract an insecure man. They both become a shallow challenge to each other. This dysfunctional relationship thrives on each one's inadequacy, -- his sense of empowerment by putting her down and controlling her appearance, and her feeling she needs to please him even when she knows deep in her heart he is wrong. The insecure female is forced to make her appearance exactly as her man wants it. He is annoyed if she changes and especially if she makes herself attractive; he fears other men may want her. His deficient manliness is not up for this challenge. A secure man is happiest when his woman is content and he is certain she will be faithful to him. There are women who come to the salon talking about what their man likes and dislikes, regardless of what makes them happy. In these cases, she sets herself up for a let-down while he gets pleasure out of seeing her miserable while trying to please his empty soul. Ask yourself why do I allow my lover to dictate how I will wear my hair? Do I dictate his hair cut?

Family and friends

Family and friends can hurt you the most. All clients who return to the salon to say they no longer like the hair-do they loved 24 hours ago have been told how ugly they look by husbands, boyfriends, grandmothers, parents, friends, etc. Unfortunately, the most cruel and harsh comments about beauty are said by "loved ones." Why do loved ones feel they have the right to hurt another's feelings by making ill intended remarks about hair texture or hair style?

In many cases they don't intend to hurt your feeling but because of familiarity they believe they have the right to control how you should look or feel they can say any-thing to you even if it is based on their own self hate and insecurity. When black women wear non-European hair styles, they are striking out, being different, and people often denigrate what's different.

What these detracting family and friends are doing is stealing happiness and good energy. They gain power by their ability to make someone else feel bad. They know it is easiest to do to someone who is a little unsure of herself. It is as if they can't stand to see anyone feel radiant and beautiful. Don't be zapped by this. Cut it off when it happens. Relatives and friends don't know they are doing it unless you tell them. Only you can let your dearest know that you will not tolerate their negative remarks and ignorant opinions. Become independent by paying for your own beauty care; that way they won't feel they have bought the right to hurt your feelings or control your hair style.

Another way to help your loved ones mind their own business is to help them recog-nize the basis for their ideals of beauty and that the world does not revolve around their concept of what is beautiful and what is not. Perhaps they have a suggestion but don't know how to give it. I have felt the need to suggest or recommend a more pleasing hair style for women who look unkempt (frizzy, frayed, soiled and slovenly styled). However, suggestions and recommendations are different from cruel remarks.

Insecure husbands and boyfriends will always feel the need to remark about any change in their woman's appearance, especially if she is looking attractive. And this thing with black men wanting to run their fingers through straight hair is a sick fantasy to have a black woman with the attributes of a Madison Avenue model. That's their problem, not yours. If they want "bouncing and behaving" hair, tell them to straighten their own hair. Or better yet, "educate" them to appreciate the beauty and softness of your natural hair.

Grandmothers, bless their hearts, and pray that they stop making you feel that you are untouched by beauty "lest your hair be straighten." This kind of woman grew up in an era when straight hair was a "green card" to the American dream. You must tell them that times have changed and it is okay to love your God-given hair texture, whether you braid it, lock it or Afro it.

As for girlfriends, there are those who love us and then there are friends who are girls. Real girlfriends who truly love you will not hurt your feelings with nasty remarks about your natural hair. Then there are co-workers and acquaintances who sometimes get too friendly. Your hair style is your personal business and should not be the subject for office conversations. For that surprise, throw-you-off-guard negative comment by such people, have a responsible come-back. Although it's not always best to go down to their level, I have found that a prepared remark will help them see their ugly ways. For example, when you go into the office with your newly braided hair style and your co-worker comments "I don't like braids," politely say, "Although I have not liked your hairdo, I never thought it was my place to tell you." I have found if you turn the tables on rude insensitive people, they usually don't want to discuss it any further. It's unfortunate you have to prepare yourself for nasty remarks disguised as concern, but it will bring you peace of mind and keep people out of your hair!

Bridal bitches

What is wrong with these women who think they can control how other women wear their hair to weddings? The audacity and nerve of these inconsiderate women! If another (grown) woman comes into my salon telling me that she can't wear her hair natural, braided or twisted to a wedding, I am going to scream. This is crazy, and I don't know who is the bigger fool, the one I call "the bridal B" or the woman trying to please her.

Let's remember a wedding is a celebration, where two people are joined by marriage. It should be festive, enjoyable, and a collective effort. I tell my clients, "Your hair texture and style have absolutely nothing to do with it. Usually you pay for the gown, shoes and other expenses to be in the wedding, and then you are insulted by some inconsiderate wedding queen who wants you to change the texture and style of your hair for the sake of her day to be in charge?"

Friends and family members are both guilty of this stupid nonsense. A daughter of one of my clients did not want her mom to come to her wedding with natural hair. She insisted that her mom straighten her natural hair. The mother, all stressed out, wanted to come very early to have her beautiful afro hair perfectly straightened for the afternoon wedding and offered an exorbitant amount to have it done. It bothered me to think a daughter could put her mother through this ordeal and the mother allow it!

Another client told me about a friend's wedding she was in and how the bride hinted to her to straighten her two-inch Afro so that the baby's breath flowers would stay in her hair. Does that make sense? Two inches of straight hair to hold baby's breath flowers? This bride was so obsessed about having all her bride's maids wear straight hair that she didn't think about how stupid she sounded suggesting that flowers will hold better in two inches of straight hair than in the soft, tight curls of a natural.

The client with the two-inch Afro told her friend she was not changing her hair and that she would be more than happy to just come to the wedding, she did not have to be in it. To make a long story short, she wore her Afro with the baby's breath flowers and was the most beautiful bridesmaid in the wedding party. So the next time you are asked to participate in someone's wedding and she tells you how to wear your hair, politely let her know you are not going to change your hair and that you do not need to be in the wedding. Don't participate in that stupidity. Hold onto your self-esteem.

What's self esteem got to do with it?

I have often seen women who are sloven, unclean, with dirty fingernails, nasty teeth, uncombed hair, body odor, and just downright disgraceful. Why don't they take better care of themselves? Why don't they notice these things? Why don't they want to feel and look better? I don't have all the answers, but I have discovered a few reasons while trying to understand this problem. They include personality, lack of knowledge, sickness (addictions, mental and emotional illness), laziness, and low or no self-esteem.

Maybe it's personality. Personalities can vary from perfectionist to the natural born slob. Lack of knowledge is surely understandable, too; we are all learning and growing. If a woman is not taught good hygiene, we can not expect her to know. Sickness, I believe can be helped and treated; we just have to extend a helping hand. Now, laziness, I haven't quite figured out. I want to yell, "Get your o#x!*'~ butt up and make yourself presentable!" Esteem seems to be linked to all or most of these in some way.

Self-esteem has come into vogue as a key element in getting the best out of life for yourself. Let's examine what it means. The dictionary definition of esteem includes the following: to set high value, respect, admire, adore, show honor and devotion; favorable opinion. Perhaps it is safe to say a woman who would neglect herself is suffering from low to no self esteem. She does not value herself enough to adore or care for her health and beauty. This unfavorable feeling about herself can lead her into a dark, confused, depressing existence.

An occasional lapse of insecurity is normal. Nobody is perfect; however, when this state consumes you every day, that becomes a problem. There is no single reason or cause for developing low self esteem. In some cases, it results from a combination of hard luck and evil influences. So what do we do? We know low self esteem negatively affects one's decisions, actions, motivation and judgment, so if we can change a woman's opinion and respect for herself, we may be able to influence her judgment and actions. If we help a woman develop a positive and loving sense of self, in all likelihood she will clean herself up and take pride in her appearance. Her body, her health and beauty will be worthy of her time and attention.

If you think you need to increase your self-esteem, start by taking small steps toward getting to know and love your spirit and body. Find all the good in yourself and thank God for the marvelous blessings. So what if you don't have a automobile, you have two healthy legs to stand on. And if your hair is not long, find the blessing in having some. Some people don't. If you don't have a job, find something you like to do; volunteer, keep yourself busy even if there's no money and simply thank God for another blessed day. Count yourself lucky not to be in a war torn country where going to work is impossible even if you wanted to. Add up your blessings and concentrate on the good in your life. We can all find some good in living.

As much as I may try, I cannot give you the powerful benefits of high self esteem. You will earn this once you capitalize on your own self worth. Remember, positive self esteem is a birthright. Find it within.

Beauty appreciation and positive thinking exercise

Are you a woman who feels defeated, constantly complains and finds the bad in everything? If yes, this makes you less ready and receptive to the beauty around you (i.e., nature, and people). Not appreciating the air we breathe or the fact that we have been blessed with another day of life means overlooking some basic things that can make life more worthwhile. No one wants to be around a person with an ugly attitude and negative vibes. With this kind of thinking and energy you will eventually come to not even appreciate yourself.

Positive thoughts will create positive results. Begin with a new attitude that will bring positive energy, good people and peacefulness to you. You are what you think and you will become what you imagine today. Take some time to yourself and notice all the marvelous things around and within you.

1. Become conscious of all people and concentrate on only the good and beautiful things about them. Even tell them how you feel about their beauty.

2. Make a list of all the things you find special about yourself.

Self Analysis Workbook

I heartily agree that "beauty is in the eye of the beholder," but the woman must first behold herself as beautiful. Beauty is more than what the eye can see. I believe beauty begins within the mind, spirit and heart. How you feel about yourself will always surface through your physical appearance. The goal of self analysis is to improve the image inside your head.

The objective of a self analysis exercise is to break down the elements that make you the person you are. For starters, look at all the hair-related events that have taken place in your life, both current and past. You can gain some understanding of why these things happened and how they have shaped your self image. Your response to these questions should be honest and spontaneous.

1. My most memorable childhood hair experience is

_____
_____
_____
_____

2. When I was growing up "good hair" was described as

_____
_____
_____
_____.

3. Three things I like most about my hair are
    a.
    b.
    c.

4. My mother says my hair is

_____

My dad says my hair is

_____.

My companion likes my hair

_____

5. When I damaged my hair, I learned

_____
_____
_____.

6. My parent/ guardian(s) were:

        nurturing, domineering, intimidating, interrogating,
        unaffectionate, liberally supportive, absent, affectionate

7. My biggest problem with hair is?

_____

_____

8. My natural hair is:

        alluring, wonderful, soft, easy, fantastic, beautiful, sexy, youthful,
        rich looking, marvelous, fine, magnetic, funky, regal

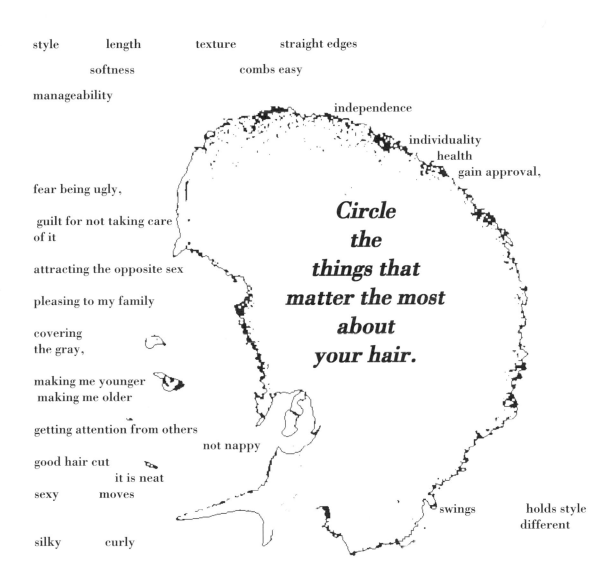

style   length   texture   straight edges

softness   combs easy

manageability

independence

individuality
health
gain approval,

fear being ugly,

guilt for not taking care of it

attracting the opposite sex

pleasing to my family

covering the gray,

making me younger
making me older

getting attention from others

not nappy

good hair cut
it is neat

sexy   moves

swings   holds style
different

silky   curly

Circle the things that matter the most about your hair.

Your answers will help you to see yourself and your hair needs.

Your lost and found

The salon is a place for "fixin' up," but you must do some personal inside work, outside of the salon. Inside beauty is inherently yours, it's simply a matter of regular self inventory to discover and nurture your personal strengths. A marvelous feeling occurs when you realize that you were born beautiful and that your natural soft, manageable kinky hair is alluring. It is an ecstatic, exciting experience for a woman to find balance, peace and beauty within herself.

Imagine how wonderful it can be to evolve from an insecure, bruised woman, to love yourself in a way that you never had before. This beauty evolution can only begin on the inside. The "Journey Within" yourself is the foundation for all the physical primping and fluffing you do to feel good. Once you have dug deep down inside yourself and pulled out the weeds, your level of consciousness can bloom while your spirit flowers. The reality of your potential as a beautiful black woman will be set in motion.

You will explore beautiful hair styles, diagnose your attributes and at this point we both will be aware of the internal and external pressures, so together we can create a style that will make you feel good about yourself first and appeal to an "appreciative audience" second. With this approach we not only strengthen your hair but your inner beauty as well.

Stop procrastinating today!

Don't let another day go by where you put off taking care of yourself. Get your rotten teeth fixed, find out why you are balding, remove your chipped, cruddy nail polish, start a health exercise regimen, (a walk will do), get your hair conditioned and anything else that you have ignored or put off for too long.

What you think will affect how you value your health and beauty and ultimately when and how to do something for it. The mind puts things into action, so don't neglect yourself. Don't allow yourself to become vulnerable and a victim of your own apathy. Self neglect is often an excuse for inadequacies and low self worth. So stop making excuses to neglect yourself! Write an urgent "to do" list. List three things concerning your health and beauty that you have put off for too long and work on it now!

1. _____

2. _____

3. _____

You are a natural beauty

Your sense of style should be based on developing a total look that works best for you rather than the latest fads or trends. One of the first steps in developing your own style is to accept that you are always learning, changing and constantly trying to find what best suits your personality and lifestyle. As you mature and become more acquainted with yourself, expect your beauty needs to change and don't be afraid of that.

Surrender to your realities and find solutions so that you don't spend time on what may appear to be problems. Sometimes we are looking for answers but we do not know the questions. What style truly makes me feel good? How am I different today than 10 years ago? Why am I never happy with my appearance? What can I afford? Although all women have the potential to be a natural beauty, many would hesitate to say that they feel this way. Human differences and the trend of unnatural lifestyles have forced an unnatural sense of being.

A natural beauty is a woman who is at her optimum wellness. She has mastered the natural process of feeling healthy and beautiful. Some women are natural-born beauties who never forget, while others have to reclaim that birthright and work at maintaining it. There are no definitive standards for natural beauty beyond cleanliness, a peaceful spirit, and an overall pleasing whole being. Whether it is the inviting smile, radiant skin, twinkle in the eyes or glowing aura, the natural beauty will know and feel when she is at this stage. Anyone who crosses her path will feel it as well.

Now that you have taken a look deep inside yourself, it should be easy to separate what is real and what is not; release the parts that are no longer worthwhile, and cultivate and make the good visible. It's time to clean house, and get rid of the beauty myths, such as "nappy hair is hard to comb," "Afro hair is ugly," and "straight hair is better." Get over the fears you have adopted, such as "I won't be able to get a job, a man or the American dream unless I change my hair." Become pro-active in your health and beauty and take control of your happiness. Share the message with those who are open to it.

Throw away the China doll wig you have hidden in your closet. Clean out all those stale hair products that are cluttering your bathroom shelves. Put a full length mirror in your bath or bedroom. Wash your hair, let it air dry and take a walk on the wild side. Get rid of the negative conditioning you have been carrying around inside yourself and take a fanciful journey for your well being.

You're on your way. God bless you.

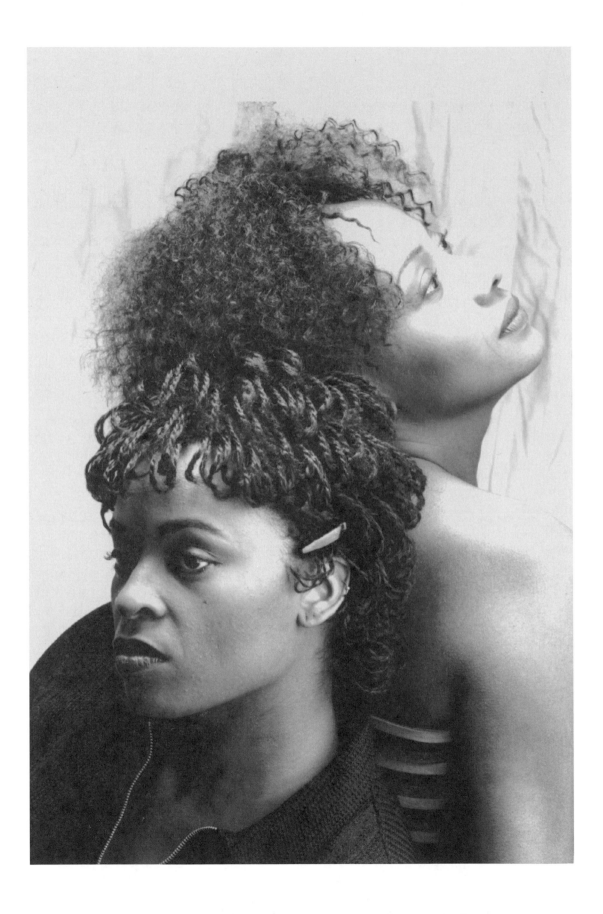

Why Grow Natural Now...

3

"I think back to when I perm my hair and realize how crazy I was. I would go to the beauty parlor at 7:30 a.m. even though the salon did not open until 9 and the stylist may come in at 9:30, 10; whenever he felt like it. Several other women and I would come to camp out early to be the first to get service; or risk having to wait until 3 p.m. Even if I was the first to be serviced, I still may not get out of the salon until 5 or 6 p.m. for a service that normally takes two hours.

The stylist never consulted with me about my style. He would say, "Chile, just sit down, I am a beautician not a magician." He would intimidate clients the moment they came in, so I avoided questioning about style or even requesting to have the burning perm rinsed out, to save myself from embarrassment. I was so simple-minded I would do this every month, never pack a lunch, be sitting in that salon hungry, tired but so desperate to get my hair fixed. And to top that, for the next two weeks I would be picking scabs from my head from the relaxer burns."
Matthews 1994

Sound familiar? It's a too-common story told by women who have stooped so low as to allow themselves to be mistreated by hair stylists and abused by themselves. Some black women really believe that the chemical hair relaxer should burn. Intelligent, educated women will sit in the beauty salon with their scalps on fire and not complain. However, if you were to put caustic lye on their new car or new silk dress, they would be ready to fight you. But their scalps, it's okay, this is normal to them.

In spite of painful episodes and the dreadful visit to the salon every month, many a black woman faithfully continues to get her hair "fixed." She rationalizes that if it does not burn, the relaxer isn't taking. She does not give any thought to the fact that the beautician wears gloves to apply this burning chemical to the hair and that there's no glove to protect her scalp. She ignores the fact that the manufacturer gives an itty bitty warning on the side of the jar, but does not include the many risks involved. It's sort of like the disclaimer on the side of a pack of cigarettes: "Do this at your own risk," is the warning. People who ignore these warnings refuse to accept that harm will come to them. It's all a part of an addiction.

And perhaps for the woman who drinks alcohol, smokes cigarettes and does drugs, it won't much matter to her if she puts a little sodium hydroxide on her scalp. However, some women go overboard into compulsive, addictive, abnormal behavior when it comes to their hair. Such a woman runs from salon to salon looking for a quick fix; has lost her hair on several occasions and has grown it back only to do it all over again. She will perm her hair one day, color it the next, recolor it, cut it short, braid it long, weave it, glue it, press the kink, all in the course of one month. What some women will do to try and feel beautiful.

It's sad to hear women who are compulsive and addicted needing a "fix" for their hair, preach about drug abusers and how they need to get help. These "preachers" need to be in a HAA (Hair Abuse Anonymous) group themselves. We all may have a little to learn about addictions. If you think you don't need HAA, stop now go cold turkey and don't ever straighten, color, perm, weave or chemically process your hair again. Ever. Many women can not do it. They will sneak, lie, deny, procrastinate, connive, run out for a no-lye relaxer, buy "Rio" from a TV ad, beg for a natural perm and do whatever they can to eliminate the kink. Or they may admit to really like relaxing their hair even though they know the process does not feel good, burns like the dickens, causes scabs, and weakens the hair. They even risk putting it on their babies heads.

Some women will even say in defense "I'm not a hair abuser or addicted to straight hair, this is my choice," Well, we all make choices and surely have the God given right to do so. What I want you to realize is that you can make choices that are more healthy. Not I nor anyone else can do this for you. You must come to this conclusion yourself. Once you realize this, you will have taken the first step toward dealing with this problem of disliking your natural hair and abusing it as a solution.

The concept of a seven-step program for the "hair abuser" follows a pattern similar to treatment for other addictions. I know this seems quite humorous, but hair abuse is a real and serious problem for some women. Many women feel helpless when it comes to loving their natural hair. And even though chemically straightening the hair has not worked for them they keep doing it because they feel too dependent to stop.

I usually ask clients who come to my salon with extremely damaged hair -- Why do you keep straightening your hair? The reasons my clients cite for continuing to straighten their hair fall under three categories:

1. **_"I'm afraid I'll mess up or sweat out my hair style."_**

Black women have changed their lifestyles to accommodate and preserve their straight hair styles. Afraid of sweating out those coiffed hairdos, these women avoid exercise, hot baths, guys with convertible cars and a strong summer breeze. Mothers have instilled this fear in their daughters. The relaxer-perm offers security; even though the style may not stay in place, the absence of the kink does. Heat pressing and blow-drying provide a temporary, physical change that is subject to perspiration, shower steam, humidity and precipitation. Even if a woman has a personal distaste for chemical applications, if she prefers straightened smooth European hair styles, she may not want the maintenance and hassle of protecting heat-pressed or blow-dried hair styles from the elements. Therefore, she resorts to chemically relaxing her hair. It becomes a permanent solution to her kinky hair.

2. **_"My beautician made me do it."_**

As I have shown in the Battle of the naps, the beautician has one goal in mind for the black woman's hair ---- make it straight and remove the nap. Some women have confided that they have been ridiculed, badgered and chastised by their beautician for not straightening their hair. Frustrated, defeated and worn down, the woman eventually gives into the beautician's demand that the only way her hair can be styled is to straighten it. When clients request services other than straightening, beautician's are at a loss because they lack the knowledge and skill to work with natural African-American hair. Such beauticians will, of course, encourage their clients to have their hair permanently straightened in order to make their job easier.

3. **_"Natural hair is not for me."_**

African-American women have expressed deep-rooted, negative sentiments about their natural hair texture. "I hate my frizzy, coily, beady, nappy hair. My hair is not pretty and it's hard to comb." "Natural styles are just not for me. When my hair is processed I feel better." Some women see their natural nap as a birth defect and would rather have thin, short, broken off, non-growing straightened hair rather than a head full of kinky hair because natural hair is not appealing to them. I am frequently asked by women "How can I go natural and still have straight hair?" It seems to me the real question is "are you really ready to go natural?"

Some women are afraid, some have found it difficult to find a stylist who will work with their natural hair, and some like their straightened hair styles too much to change. There are women who will chemically process their hair until the day they die, and I am not here to change that. There are also women who are not ready to give up straight styles forever, but occasionally want to give their hair a rest from using hot irons, rollers or chemical hair products. These can be times when a woman is pregnant and decides to not put chemicals on her scalp while carrying the fetus, or when she wants to wear a simple style that will allow her hair to grow, or she is interested in summertime hair care that will work well at the beach. All this is possible with natural styling, braids and even natural hair weaves to cover and give any hair a rest.

As an alternative to chemically processing the hair to achieve wavy, curly or straight textures, a hair weave can be worn for a temporary texture and style change. If you want a wavy or krimpy texture, add hair extension to protect your hair rather than altering it. Done by a skilled braider, these natural styling options allow you to try new hair styles with no permanent commitment and no risk of hair damage.

Whether you choose to go natural forever or just need to give your chemically-processed hair a natural rest, knowing what's available gives you the power to be pro-active and not re-active to your hair needs. It is better to do this because you want to, not because you have to. Some women who prefer to chemically process their hair plan every six months to give their hair a natural rest. Others eventually find a natural style that replaces their need to chemically process the hair. Both benefit by making wise decisions for healthy hair care.

Are you a "hair abuser?"

If you recognize yourself as a hair abuser and feel your hair problems are consuming too much of your time and happiness, seek through prayer the answer to what you should do with your hair. Follow this plan:

° Ask for guidance from God to remove your sense of shortcomings.
° Look in the mirror and recite your Seven Step Affirmation. (see pg. 48)
° Look for a hair care stylist who works with natural hair and is supportive.

The best way to find a hair care stylist is to ask women with healthy hair where they get their hair done and the name of their stylist. Find out how long they have been going to that stylist and if they are really satisfied. Call the salon and ask to have a brief consultation with this stylist. This is necessary because you need to talk with someone who understands that you are going through a transition and trying to simplify your life and hair care regimen. Once you become aware and pray for guidance, you will meet many women of like mind and with healthy hair. This is not by coincidence; this is receiving the energy from where your attention is focused. You must ask the question before you can get the answers.

Seek a hair care stylist who will condition and style your hair in a simple style that requires minimal fuss and upkeep. The idea is to liberate yourself from impulses to do something harmful to your hair. Free yourself from half a day's work on your head. Work on simplicity and healthy hair. Look for a salon that is peaceful, intimate and unhurried. In this salon environment, you are not easily tempted to try the latest fad or to relapse.

A natural hair support group

A support group can be a great benefit because it consists of people like yourself. It is an opportunity to exchange ideas, techniques, and information that will be helpful and encouraging. Many times there are personal and emotional matters women may want to discuss about their hair but family or friends don't understand and traditional salons are not trained to offer these services, so it is a lot easier to talk to someone who has gone through the process.

Women who are suffering hair loss from medication, or an illness that affects the hair, are relieved to talk to someone who is going through the same situation. In the group meetings the discussions can include how women have coped, what things they used to help their problem, alternative hair care and styling options that otherwise are not offered in salons.

One kind of support group rather than a therapy session, is an information workshop to ask questions and get advice on how other women have overcome their hair problems. You can start a support group in your area that is general or specific, such as support for women who have husbands who hate their hair, women who are going natural, women who are balding, who are obsessed with long straight hair, etc.

To organize a support group in your area, you can start with as few as three people and seek someone who is knowledgeable about hair care with leadership abilities to keep the discussion going and provide correct information. Ask a local hair care person to lead a session to get you started. Post an ad in a local health food store, exercise gym or braid salon that is specific about the kind of group you would like to form or attend. Hair abuse and hair related problems often are not viewed as serious problems, they are often trivialized and treated as purely cosmetic. However, there are women whose low self esteem is triggered by hair problems. I have seen the psychological, emotional and physical wounds and I know that healing is more important and deeper than a fancy hairdo.

Unfortunately, there are no national hotlines or trained volunteers women can call when they feel weak and desperate for advice. The best resources are people who understand the problem and a professional hair care stylist who has the insight to help your specific need.

Seven-Step Affirmation

Repeat aloud:

1. I admit I am never satisfied with my hair; I am out of control. I have lost the self-discipline to stop doing things to my hair that are harmful and unhealthy.

2. I will have faith in God's will, accept that God makes no mistakes and that my hair texture is not a mistake; it is beautiful and in the image of God.

3. I will get to know myself, accept who I am and in prayer, be thankful for my good health and growing hair.

4. I will become informed, knowledgeable, and practice my own healthy hair care. I will seek support, guidance and a loving plan to care for my hair.

5. I will no longer negate my innate beauty, nor participate in negative remarks, jokes, and comments about other women's hair.

6. I will instill in my children self pride, teach them to appreciate their natural hair, and I will always speak lovingly about their natural beauty.

7. I will practice self preservation, self love, and value God's beauty. My hair care will be based on good health and honesty.

Feeling weak

The worse time to go to a new salon is during a moment of desperation. This is when you are the most vulnerable. A good hair care stylist who knows you, and you are more to her than a meal ticket, will not give service that is not needed or that could be detrimental and morally wrong. For example, if you go to a salon and you are clearly bald on the sides and in the crown, you just put in a home perm yesterday, and you ask a beautician to color your hair blond because you have a dance to attend tonight and you are willing to pay double if she squeezes in your appointment --watch out! Many unscrupulous and unknowing beauticians will jump at the opportunity to make the "money." They will not think twice about your hair condition and desperate disposition. The conscientious beautician, however, will say "no," because this will ruin your hair. Instead, she will give you some other options. You may not like it at that moment, but it will prove to be the best decision for your hair.

Often in the heat of desperation, women don't realize what they ask for. They request things they don't need. If you get a desperate urge to do anything to your hair, take a long walk, then shampoo, condition, and pull your hair back neatly and wear a beautiful hat or head wrap. Cover up until you can decide on a style at a more self-assured time. Most women abuse and ruin their hair at their low, desperate, and vulnerable moments. And the uncaring beauticians see you coming. Perhaps if she doesn't do it, you'll do it anyway. Self control is the solution.

You may relapse

I am always relieved and joyful when I influence a woman's decision to stop putting chemicals on her scalp, especially if she comes to the salon with extremely damaged hair. The more I see grown women who are struggling with this "hair thing," I understand that some women will constantly feel guilty about it. Some women learn after going bald once that chemical hair care is not good for them. They make a conscious decision to go natural and there is no turning back. Unfortunately, more women do not learn the lessons and do not believe the damage could happen again.

I expect women to get weak and relapse. It's a part of the transition and fight with addiction to hair abuse; to keep repeating the same compulsive behavior, a behavior that is temporarily fulfilling. If this sounds like you, don't give up on yourself. Even though you may feel like you are taking one step forward and two steps backward, you are at least aware of your behavior. The turning point is when you discover why you keep doing it and I hope this will help you resist the temptation to continue this compulsive behavior.

Lack of knowledge

Ignorance and lack of information are the greatest causes for hair problems. In some cases women know and have experienced what works and what does not work on their hair, but they choose to ignore this. On the other hand many women have been told all the wrong things about their hair. They've been brainwashed into thinking curly hair does not grow long, or is dry and will break if it isn't permed. They've been told that kinky hair is unmanageable, needs straightening, is too hard to comb, and so on.

The lack of correct and sensible information has sent the black woman on a road of misguided hair care. Some women have gone bald in the process, worn hairdos they hate, and have done things to their hair that they regret. Yet they continue to navigate in the dark and seek the wrong solutions for their hair care needs. The simplest grooming tips often seem to be the most difficult to find, and knowledgeable beauticians are few and desperately sought after.

The wide selection of cosmetics and hair products available, however, give many women the false sense that they are knowledgeable and skilled. Go into any beauty supply store usually owned and operated by non-cosmetologists and you can get a five-minute lesson on how to relax, color or bleach your precious strands of hair. No license is needed, just the time, money and willingness to experiment on your own hair. Even though most hair chemical product labels say "for professional use only," any 12-year-old child can go into a drug store and purchase a relaxer kit, or a frustrated, unthinking mother can apply "kiddy perm" to her baby's curly tresses. Black women risk problems when they try to care for their hair in the absence of sound information that relates to it.

Hair products and harmful chemicals that can be applied by untrained and unthinking people are more easily found than a trained and knowing beautician. Today any beautician can count on one hand the number of students in her cosmetology class who understood the structure of black women's hair, chemistry and anatomy.

The 1990s black woman is not as fortunate as our grandmothers were. The black cosmetologists in those days cared about their clients' hair. These were the beauticians of the "old school." Ask any elder woman whose hair grew for 50 years until she started going to the modern young beautician who chemically treated her natural hair. More elder women are balding at the hands of young uncaring beauticians than ever before. The "old school" hair dresser would question new styles and services that were risky and dangerous to the hair follicle. They were honored, reliable, and in some cases more valuable than the doctor. Many of today's hair stylists are more interested in making money. And you, the desperate consumer, are their dollar sign.

You must take the necessary precautions and sensible steps to become aware of your hair and the products you put on it. And, yes, there are some beauticians who frown upon educating the consumer for fear of losing clients; however, I think we all have something to gain if we are working toward the same objective -- healthy, beautiful hair. I realize that black women have searched for a solution to styling and grooming their curly textured hair and have resorted to chemicals because natural care has been most difficult to find. Healthy hair care is about taking charge of your own hair and becoming an educated consumer, so that the braider or stylist you select will care for your hair like you would. Hair care starts with you.

Let's talk about different hair conditions.

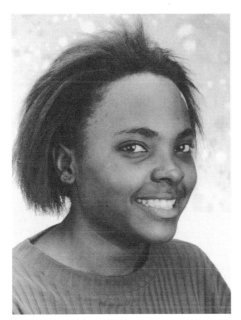

1. Relaxed hair

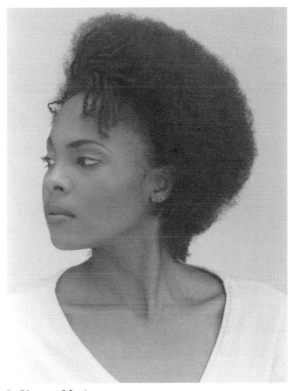

2. Natural hair

The two photos are the same person. (1) Relaxed hair two years prior to (2) all natural hair, chemical free.

There are differences between the hair in its natural state and when you physically and or chemically style it. We will briefly discuss these hair conditions to get an absolute basic understanding of your hair state and condition.

Virgin (natural) hair

Virgin hair is your God-given natural hair texture, in the original condition as it grows from the follicle. Hair comes in many different textures -- curly, wavy, straight, and kinky, textures formed by the shape of your hair follicle. The black woman's natural hair is beautiful, soft, responsive and manageable. It's easy to care for, particularly when the right products and correct combing methods are used.

Any hair that has been chemically altered (i.e., by relaxers, permanent waves, curly perms, hair colors) is no longer in its virgin condition; it is considered un-natural. There are no products, solutions, or cosmetic procedures that will reverse the chemically altered hair back to its original texture or color. You will have to grow new hair and cut away the chemically treated hair.

Neglected virgin hair has been uncared for or improperly handled. This results from infrequent shampoos, harsh combing, and suffocating the hair follicle with unnatural products (grease, gels, sprays, activators, etc.). The problem occurs also if the hair is never conditioned or is groomed with products formulated for opposing hair types. These things can cause curly natural hair to feel hard, look dull, tangle and become uneven from breakage at the ends. After years, even generations, of this mistreatment, no wonder people have come to believe virgin hair is unmanageable.

Relaxed hair

The relaxer is a process to chemically straighten curly hair. It permanently changes the characteristics of naturally curly, kinky hair textures. Correctly relaxed hair is slightly straightened without completely removing the curl. This relaxed hair is strong and does not show any areas of breakage, baldness or thinning. The texture, although chemically altered, is not extremely contrasting to the natural hair texture, and if conditioned regularly and relaxed no more than three times a year, will feel healthy. Hair that is not over relaxed is the easiest to grow out because the relaxed ends and the new growth are not dramatically different.

Over relaxed hair is over-processed and has been over-exposed to chemicals, causing the ends to become fragile and break easily. The hair can also fall out or thin throughout areas of the head. The use of strong hair dyes and hair relaxers dissolve areas of the cuticle, leaving the weakened hair more susceptible to damage. Damaged hair can be recognized by signs

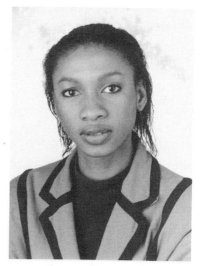

Over-processed relaxed hair

of white, brittle, split ends, matting and tangling while wet, and feeling coarse and stiff when dry. The hair does not style or curl easily.

Relaxed beyond repair hair is the worst condition for hair, besides baldness. When the hair is in this condition it is not worth keeping, and one can only hope for fast new growth in order to cut the ends off to start fresh. This hair is completely ruined from harsh chemical solutions which cause it to look sparse, and limp when wet, and brittle when dry. Often, sparse pieces of the relaxed hair are left while the breakage is as short as 1/8". Hair in this condition may be too fragile to comb, style and handle.

Chemical hair relaxer

The active ingredient in hair relaxer is sodium hydroxide (a caustic soda lye) or ammonium thioglycolate. The FDA banned the use of more than 10 percent of this lye in household liquid drain cleaners, because the lye will corrode drain pipes. It is a strong alkaline with a PH of 14. Because it is very strong, it may cause dermatitis of the scalp. If left on the hair more than 10 minutes, it will dissolve the hair, causing it to tear easily and become fragile and limp. Frequent and strong inhalation of this chemical can lead to lung damage.

Permed hair

The curly perm is a chemical process that straightens then re-curls naturally curly hair. It is better known as the "curl." Usually the processed hair is moistened with an activator product that coats the hair with oil and other chemicals to maintain the wet curl. If the hair is over-processed it becomes thin and limp on the ends with very short breakage down to the new growth. Sometimes the new growth is like a short Afro with sprigs of fragile permed hair hanging on.

Cold wave

The permanent cold wave is a chemical application to make naturally straight hair wavy and curly. This style is quite popular with Caucasians. It is different than the "curl" because it is a one-process chemical and does not require heat to make it work; thus, it is called the cold wave. It processes at room temperature and has a PH level of 9.6. The straight hair is set on perm rollers and the perm solution of thioglycolic acid, ammonia, sometimes borax, ethanolamine or sodium lauryl sulfate is applied to the hair. After the processing time, it is neutralized to lock in the new permanent curl. The neutralizer chemicals consist of sodium or potassium bromate, hydrogen peroxide or sodium perborate. If the solution is not rinsed thoroughly and is done frequently, it, too, can cause hair thinning and hair loss. If straight hair is over processed it will become frizzy and dry. "The thioglycolates are toxic and may cause skin irritation and low blood sugar. Among injuries recently reported to the FDA were hair damage, swelling of the legs and feet, eye irritation, rash in area of ears, necks, scalp and forehead, and swelling of the eyelids."[4]

Chemical curly perm

The permanent curl, and the cold wave are both chemicals that are used on rodded hair to create a curl. However the curl is processed with heat and is a double chemical application. The hair is in double jeopardy because it is first chemically straightened with sodium hydroxide, rolled on perm rods, then another chemical (thio) is applied. Next, sodium perborate is applied to neutralize the acids that curled the hair, then the client is placed under a hot hair dryer for at least an hour. Thus, the scalp, which has already been traumatized by the chemicals, is further distressed by heat. Thioglycolic acid compounds are used in the chemical solution.

The greatest danger in using this process is the risk of a chemical burn on the crown of the scalp. A chemical burn will cause scarring of the tissue. Hair cannot grow through scarred tissue because the follicles are closed by the hardened skin. This is probably what causes the male pattern balding you see in women who have worn the curly perm to long. The scalp looks shiny and the skin is tight and cracked.

Dye, lighten and colored hair

Chemically removing the natural color from hair is done through a process known as bleaching or lightening. Some of the chemicals found in hair lighteners are hydrogen peroxide, ammonia, ammonium hydroxide, and sodium peroxide. The ammonia has a tendency to strip the hairs natural oils, causing the hair to become dry, coarse and brittle. The ends are noticeably split and break easily in the brush or comb. To avoid over exposure, never use a dye with another chemical process, such as a perm or relaxer.

Permanent hair color

Hair can be colored by adding a vegetable, metallic, oxidation dye or tint color deposit. To permanently change the natural color, hydrogen peroxide is used with the hair color. Many beauticians use a permanent color method with a 20-40 volume hydrogen peroxide to open the cuticle layer, allowing the color to seep into the pigment layer of the hair and to make hair color more intense and long lasting. Usually, if there are two bottles to be mixed together, this it is a permanent hair color. This process can cause the hair to become coarse and dry. Numerous studies have shown that coal tar hair dyes are mutagenic and potentially carcinogenic.

Heat press

A hot steel comb heated at a very high temperature is applied directly to the hair shaft, to straighten curly hair. Although it is not toxic like a chemical straightener, the heat press can be damaging if the hair is overly straightened and repeatedly stretched by the very hot comb and heavy hair oil. After a time, the hair ends will stretch, lose elasticity, become thin and uneven, and not revert to its natural curl. The advantage over the chemical straightener is that other than a scalp burn from the hot comb, no chemicals are absorbed through the skin.

Both chemical processing and hot pressing the hair will cause split hair ends. Split ends can be found at the very end of the hair strand. They are caused from daily handling, harsh chemicals and repeated heat. If the end point is white or split like a fork, it qualifies as a split end. There is not much that can done to repair spit ends, some hair oils or conditioners may cover the split ends but the best solution is to cut them off.

Chemically over-processed hair

Many people who are applying chemicals to hair do not fully understand the application process. The correct application to avoid overprocessing the hair is to apply the chemical to new growth; virgin hair only. However many woman have over-processed hair because they touch-up the new growth and overlap it onto the already chemically treated hair. A "virgin relaxer" is the first-time application to natural hair; a touch-up or re-touch relaxer is to apply the chemical to the new growth hair only. Do not apply relaxer to already relaxed hair.

Once you have relaxed the hair, there is no need to re-apply relaxer. The relaxed hair cannot get any straighter, but only thinner because the chemical is melting down the protective layers of the hair shaft. Curly, kinky hair that is relaxed to silky, flimsy hair is melted down. It's like overcooked pasta; that turns into mush. Leave the relaxer or any chemical on the hair too long or apply too much and the hair will turn to a mushy, slimy texture while wet. Is your hair over-processed? Here's how you can check it and prevent it from happening. What to look for is limp, thin hair that tears easily.

Test if your hair is chemically over-processed:

1. Wet your hair thoroughly. Hold the hair midway between fingers of both hands and stretch the hair ; if the hair tears or rips easily -- something is wrong! Strong healthy hair has an elastic nature and easily stretches and returns to its original length.
2. If your hair matt's and sticks together when it is wet -- something is wrong!
3. Is your hair thin, limp and flat when wet and feels like straw and looks ashy when dry?   if yes -- something is wrong!

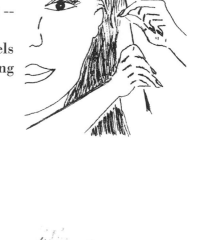

How to avoid over-processing your hair

1. Don't put chemicals on your hair in the first place, because it is next to impossible to not overlap the chemical onto the already relaxed hair.

2. If you do, make sure that during the touch-up process, the chemical is applied to the new hair only.

3. Do not leave the chemical on the hair for a long period, get touch-ups no more than three times a year and don't apply the chemical to the edges first.

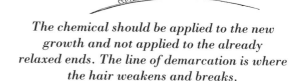

Relaxed ends

Demarcation line

New growth

The chemical should be applied to the new growth and not applied to the already relaxed ends. The line of demarcation is where the hair weakens and breaks.

What does chemical processing do to the hair?

The hair has two bonds, a physical bond (hydrogen) and a chemical bond (sulphur), referred to as the S and H bonds. Chemically processing the hair changes the molecular structure by breaking down the hairs "S" and "H" bonds. These bonds create the "S-shaped" kink or curl in African-American hair. Once the S bond is broken, the hair loses much of its natural shape and resiliency, and can be manually formed to straight hair. The changed S-shape bond can never be returned to its original curly form. It has undergone a chemical change; becoming a new shaped hair with different properties than the original hair. This is like burning wood to ash; it cannot become wood again. Once the hair has been chemically altered, it cannot revert to its curly form.

The strength or percentage of the active substance in hair chemical products should be adjusted for each person's hair texture and desired results. Unfortunately, many beauticians think that because hair is nappy or has kink, it is coarse in texture. Such errors in judgement causes the unthinking person to use too strong a chemical on the hair, which often results in over-processing and dissolving the hair.

What does all this really mean? In the wrong hands, chemicals can be dangerous. Caustic lye put onto hair is like bleach on fabric -- if left on too long it will dissolve and destroy the fibers. Sodium hydroxide and ammonium thioglycolate perm solutions are both corrosive substances that really have no place in the beauty salon. Once the hair has been relaxed or permed it is unchangeable and irreversible. If you want the original texture back, consider the relaxer or perm application like a hair cut. You will need to grow the original texture hair back.

Chemicals on your body

Chemical processing involves more than simply straightening or texturizing the hair above the scalp. Chemicals absorb through the skin into the tissue, cells and blood stream. So if you chemically process your hair on a regular basis (every four weeks) it increases your exposure to these toxic cosmetics. The real danger is the over-exposure to the chemicals; that is what increases the risk for harm. The instructions for using hair chemicals advises wearing gloves because the chemical is caustic, however it is applied directly to your hair and scalp and left there for a period of time. Why would manufacturers advise wearing gloves to protect the hands and not the scalp? And why do women experience burns and scabs if this is not harmful? Many women are exposed to these chemicals from six to 12 times a year, on an average of 15 or more years.

Even the beauticians who daily inhale these chemical vapors, have no idea of the occupational hazards they risk. Chemical solutions in salon-size bottles are not required by law to list the ingredients of that product. And very few if any salons or consumers have a MSDS (Material Safety Data Sheet) on the hair chemicals they use. If you have a reaction to a hair chemical you would not have information on the hazardous ingredients, emergency first aid advice, ways to prevent hazardous chemicals from entering the body or at least how to properly store this product.

Toxic chemicals can enter the body through the skin and lungs. It is not by chance that a high incidence of respiratory problems, lung damage and cancer is found among beauty salon personnel. Unfortunately, extensive studies have not been conducted on the health problems of African-American cosmetologists and their customers. Whose benefit would it serve? Not the hair chemical manufacturers. They give you the warning on the side of the box and the choice is yours. If you wish to exercise your freedom of choice, know the dangers and side effects. And know that you alone take responsibility for putting toxic cosmetics in your body.

Absorption of chemicals can cause disease

Noted cancer surgeon and researcher Barbara Justice, M.D., emphatically stated, "Absolutely. Positively. Chemicals which cause change in the natural physiology and biochemistry can lead to abnormal growths." She added, "The use of chemicals on the hair and scalp is physically unhealthy. As yet we have no idea of the full effect of absorption of these chemicals through the skin. However, an increasing volume of research points to the modern explosion of malignancy and other immune dysfunction diseases (i.e. rheumatory arthritis, multiple sclerosis, sarcoidosis, etc.). These malignancies are caused by the release of free-radicals into our system. Free-radicals are abnormal molecules that cause damage to the normal orderly process of the body's immune maintenance. The increase of free-radicals is believed to be caused by increased amounts of toxins and poisons in our environment which are absorbed into our body in various ways. Therefore, a case can be made that the additional load of free-radicals induced by the use of toxic hair chemicals contributes to immune depression and consequently the development of ubiquitous diseases and cancers."[5]

We know for a fact chemicals and drugs absorb into the skin. The medical industry administers drugs "transdermally," such as the arm patch, where drugs are attached to an adhesive strip to be transferred through the skin, to help people stop smoking, or for birth control and motion sickness.

To become a cosmetologist it is required that you understand the properties and functions of the outer skin (epidermis) and the underneath skin (dermis). This information is very important because it is the foundation of healthy hair care practice. I practice with the understanding that there is more to hair than what meets the eye, and that the hair shaft is truly an extension of the body, not a dead fiber that extends from the head.

The skin, including that which covers the scalp, has the function of protecting the body against harmful matter entering it and from necessary material seeping out. Its important functions -- to protect and regulate the body temperature, sensitivity, absorption, secretion, and excretion -- are all vital and should not be underestimated. The outer skin is relatively firm to protect the delicate tissues and cells underneath .

When I realized part of the requirement for becoming a licensed cosmetologist was that I would have to become proficient in applying corrosive chemicals to the hair and skin, I understood the importance of studying anatomy and chemical compositions. This was not my practice as a hair braider. Hair braiding is a natural and therapeutic process. In fact, many women would braid their hair to give it a rest from chemical damage.

My question still remains: Why put poisonous, toxic chemicals on the skin when one of its functions is absorption? It made no sense to me, because it is a violation to the body and downright dangerous, including the inhalation of these toxic fumes. I became more and more concerned that consumers trust beauticians and evidently never think they are in any danger from putting chemicals on their scalps. Perhaps some women don't care, as long as they live and die "beautiful," but there are women who are not aware because the information is not made public. Studies are rarely presented to the population that is at risk, even though they are available. Numerous studies have demonstrated the dangers related to hair dyes and other chemicals cosmetologists use daily. Several studies suggest that cosmetics used frequently, especially by cosmetologists, are carcinogenic and mutagenic. Carcinogenic means -- capable of causing cancer; mutagenic means it can cause damage to the genetic material that can affect future generations of children.

Carcinogenic risks, from chemical absorption and inhalation.

A study done by the Cancer Surveillance program at the University California School of Medicine found the number of cases of multiple myeloma (blood cancer) to be excessive for females in the occupation "cosmetologist, hairdressers, and manicurist." Dr. John Peters said in The American Journel of Industrial Medicine, that "among the suspect substances are hair dyes, shampoos, hair conditioners, relaxers, permanent wave solution, detergents, nail antiseptics, fungi and bacteria. Although the study does not account for race in the findings, blacks typically have higher rates of multiple myelomas."[6]

Numerous studies show that certain hair dyes are carcinogenic. A study reported in the American Heart Journal, found that women who dyed their hair had significantly more lymphoctic chromosomal damage than women of the same age and habits who did not.[7] These results suggested that hair dyes were penetrating the scalp and causing genotoxic effects in the lymphocytes.

Studies have shown a high incidence of asthma, lung cancer, reproductive disorders, dermatitis and other chemical sensitivities among cosmetologists. Signs of chemical storage and toxicity in the body are numbness and tingling of the fingers and hands, headaches, loss of breath, fatigue, memory loss, dizziness and aches in the body.

Because cosmetologists, and women in general, are exposed routinely to hair relaxers, hair sprays, permanent wave solutions, makeup, shampoo, conditioners, hair dyes, and nail polishes, they are at a high risk for tumors and cancers. Some of the compounds used in cosmetics are known mutagens and suspected carcinogens. Until further tests specific to the African-American female are done, it is your responsibility to protect yourself from exposure to these substances. To decrease your chances of exposure, it is best to use chemicals in moderation, if at all.

We are constantly exposed to so many external pollutants and environmental contaminant's, the least we can do is make a conscious decision to lessen the intake of toxins we put on our bodies. Natural hair care provides a healthy substitution of non-hazardous styling processes and cosmetics.

Are you protected from unsafe cosmetics?

There is a distinct difference between how the Food & Drug Administration (FDA) defines and regulates a cosmetic and a drug. A drug relieves, cures and diagnosis, whereas a cosmetic's claim or purpose is to simply improve appearance. Some products, however, are a cosmetic and a drug, such as dandruff shampoo. As a consumer you are protected by the regulation of drugs but no mandatory regulations are required for cosmetics. To regulate and protect the consumer, drug manufacturers are required by FDA law to pre-register every year and update their list of manufactured drugs two times a year, whereas cosmetic manufacturers can voluntarily register their cosmetics. They are not required by law to list the ingredients or the quantities of substances used in beauty cosmetics.

Unfortunately, a very small percent (less than 20 percent of an estimated 5,000 manufacturers) have filed ingredient statements or product experience reports. So if a cosmetic is faulty, the FDA cannot take action until it has been proven to be harmful to human beings. In 1994, a new hair straightening product called "Rio" was introduced. Subsequently, black women who used it suffered hair loss and in some instances their hair turned a green color. After numerous complaints, the FDA banned the use of the product until further study.

It is the consumer's responsibility to report problems from cosmetic products. And if the product proves to be harmful, you may have served as the unknowing test sample. Basically, until the consumer reports the problem, such as what happened with "Rio," the FDA does not have any idea of the new products that make their way to your bathroom shelves. The FDA does not approve products, it disapproves them once you report a problem with it.

Because it is voluntary for product manufacturers to report information about their products to the FDA, they tell very little, especially about the percentages of ingredients used, perhaps for fear that someone may steal their formula. The consumer is at risk because some ingredients are more dangerous based on their concentrations. For example, the FDA banned the use of more than 10 percent of sodium hydroxide in household liquid drain cleaners, but it is voluntary, not mandatory, for manufacturers of hair relaxers to report the percentage of sodium hydroxide (one of the main ingredients) in their products. Your beautician most likely does not know the percentage of sodium hydroxide in the hair relaxer used on your scalp.

Another contaminant, 1,4-dioxane, that has been shown to cause cancer can be found in emulsion-based cosmetics containing polyethylene derivatives. This, too, is an ingredient found in hair relaxers, and again, the consumers do not know the percentage used in the product formulation.

Unfortunately people do not usually suspect cosmetics of causing cancer, mutations or any disease, because we assume they are safe to use. This is not always the case. Your only safety from hazardous cosmetics is to become knowledgeable and aware of what ingredient you put on your body. It is your responsibility to police your health.

If you should experience serious problems with a cosmetic that cannot be resolved by the manufacturer, write to the

FDA Cosmetics Technology Division / Food and Drug Administration
5600 Fisher Lane
Rockville, MD 20857

Undesirable substances in frequently used hair cosmetics

1. Hair relaxer -- *sodium hydroxide, polyethlene glycol*
2. Permanent wave solution -- *Ammonium thioglycolate, alkaline sulfite, borax*
3. Shampoos -- *formaldehyde, sodium lauryl sulfate, various dyes, propylene, methyl cellulose*
4. Hair conditioners -- *glycerolstearate alcohols, stearallonium chloride, various dyes*
5. Hair Dyes -- *n-nitro-o-phenylenediamine, 4-ethoxy-m-phenylenediamine, 2,Diaminoanisole, 2,4 diaminotoluene*
6. Hair Sprays -- *Methelyne Chloride*

Grow Natural Now

Natural hair care means styling and grooming your hair without using toxic chemicals that permanently change or alter its original texture and absorb into the body. You can comb the hair into styles that enhance the natural texture while using naturally derived products formulated to keep the hair and skin healthy.

Heat-pressed or blow-dried hair is still natural because the hair is only temporarily changed. Even though a hot press can be damaging to the hair shaft over a long period of time, there is no risk of chemical absorption in the skin. The hair will return to its original texture once it's wet. Natural styling, braiding, twisting, hair locking, and barbering are healthy methods that change the hairs appearance, but do not change the hairs natural properties. Before you can enjoy natural styling you will have to grow out the chemically treated hair. *First look at your length, texture, amount of new hair growth, perm ends and overall hair condition, using the following guidelines*:

To get an idea of how much new growth you have, thoroughly wet your hair and look at the hair closest to the scalp. The new growth will be curly kinky, while the ends remain straight.

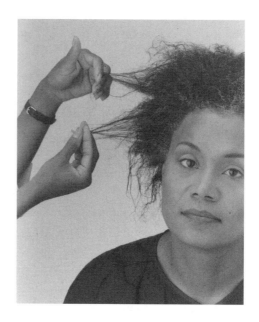

Here's how to begin growing natural hair. Once you have decided to stop relaxing and processing your hair, this section will guide you how to do it. To begin growing out hair that has been relaxed, curly permed or chemically texturized, choose a style that will make growing it out less frustrating as the hair grows out with two different hair textures. We will call this the **transition phase.** The objective is to select a transition hair style to protect the hair as it is growing out so that you don't experience any further damage or feel the temptation to process the new growing hair. The long-term goal is to grow a full head of natural healthy hair.

Making the Transition

1. Hair that is too short to braid, extremely damaged, broken off throughout, and has up to 1" of new growth should be cut off. With this hair condition, you have to cut it off or cover it up with a wig or hat for several months.

2. Hair that has at least three inches in length and is not broken in large areas can be laid to rest with a braid or weave transition style. This option will add length and volume where needed while protecting the growing hair. With the extension, you can create a "wish style" or duplicate how you were wearing your hair prior to growing natural.

3. Hair that is five inches or more without any noticeable hair breakage can be styled into a pin-up roll, bun or loose braid. If the hair textures are in great contrast, this option will only work well for several months. After that, a braid or extension style may better protect the hair.

4. For hair that is recently processed (within six weeks), fragile, overprocessed, too weak to braid and not enough new growth to cut into a short natural, cover the hair with a wig, hat or stylish head wrap. This is your only choice until you get at least 1" of new growth.

The transition style serves two purposes -- protecting the new growing hair and creating a flattering hairdo. Select a transition style that protects the hair and is suited to your hair condition. The idea is to still look beautiful and feel pretty while your hair is rejuvenating. The most challenging part will be to find the hair style that really works for your hair and lifestyle. The following four transition options are intended to guide and get you started. Some of you may feel limited in choices but as your hair begins to grow you will have many more style possibilities.

1. Cut off the chemical hair!

A quick and easy way to grow natural hair is to simply cut off all of the chemically processed hair. Have your natural stylist or barber cut off the processed ends down to the new growth hair. Since the average growth of hair on the scalp is about 1/2" per month, you may wait at least four months after the hair was chemically processed so that you will have up to two inches of new hair growth.

If you want a "natural" that is longer than two inches, you will need to wait more than four months to grow a considerable length of new hair. To be sure that the new growth is consistent throughout the head; the hair should be cut while it is wet. This allows the stylist to see the line of demarcation between the natural curly hair and the straight relaxed or chemically treated hair. To avoid straight spiky ends, cut the hair below the line of demarcation and make sure there is enough new growth throughout. If the hair is cut above the line of demarcation, it creates a spiky straight end effect. This too, however makes for an interesting style.

The short natural is a very attractive, low maintenance style for curly hair. It requires no rolling, curling or complicated daily styling other than brushing and combing. When it is cut according to your hair texture and hair type, this will bring out the true beauty in any curly texture hair. The hair texture and condition determine a potential style, but the stylist is the key to creating it. Choose a stylist who appreciates natural hair and is familiar with the many degrees of curl in African American hair. The stylist also must look for differing hair patterns and textures on one person's head.

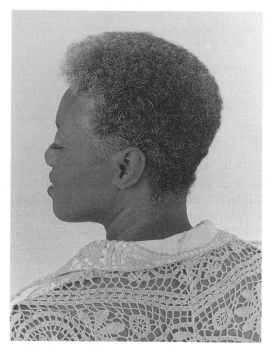

A classic short natural hair cut.

If you live in an area that does not have a great number of braiders, natural stylists, or African-American barbers, a short cut is possible by any cosmetologist or barber who is skilled in hair cutting. There are two methods of cutting the natural hair: scissor and clipper (razor) cut.

A cut done by a stylist who works well with these two methods, will have an end result that is similar. However, the scissor cut works especially well for fine, soft-textured hair and perimeter soft finishing work. With the scissor cut, the stylist has more control over a precision cut because the hair is stretched out and the curl is usually cut at the same angle, regardless of the direction you may comb it. The clipper cut may look very even to the eye, but will show uneven strands if it is done by an amateur and is combed against the direction of the clipper cut. To remove hair clippings and to check for uneven ends, have the barber stylist shampoo your hair immediately after the clipper cut.

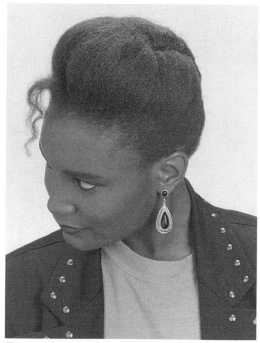

Pin-up style for long transition hair.

One complaint I often hear from women who have had their hair cut by a barber is that the style looks masculine. If you decide to have a barber cut your hair, consult with the barber first and say you do not want a severe looking cut. Ask that the hairline be left in its natural form or that the finishing be done to look soft. A clipper trim line around the front hairline and in front of the ears gives a severe hard edge effect. If the hairline permits, have the barber or stylist fade the back hairline rather than make a distinct trim line. To give softness to a short natural, scissor cut in front of the ear, leaving the hair longer and wispy thin. Never cut the front hair line. This will cause the hairline to grow back coarse and unsightly. A beautiful feminine hair cut is cut softly along the hairline to frame the face.

To ensure a flattering and attractive natural, the hair texture, head shape, facial features and curl pattern should all be considered before cutting the hair short. There are some special considerations like a flat head, small head, large head, protruding ears, receding hairline and high forehead that must be incorporated into how the hair cut will look.

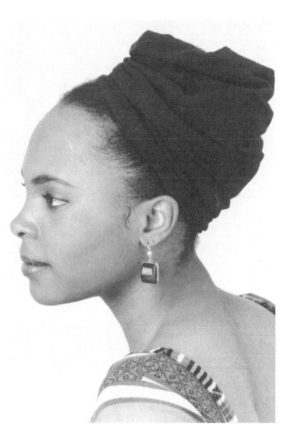

The short natural is a great option, however some women may feel uncomfortable cutting all their hair off. For hair that is extremely damaged, where more then 50 percent of the hair is broken off down to less than 2", you may be limited to a short cut, a wig or hat. If you have enough hair in reasonable condition, there are other ways to grow natural. Try one of the other style options.

2. Pin-up

Cover up with a Hair Tucker.(pg.68)

For relaxed long and straight hair that is strong enough to work with but needs a rest from heat and pulling, a pin-up stationary style is manageable. The pin-up style requires minimal combing, and no direct heat. If your chemically straightened hair is quite long and the texture difference is slight, you can continue to style the hair without the "relaxer touch up." Your beautician may try to frighten you by saying if you don't get a touch up your hair will break.

Hair that breaks from not getting a relaxer touch up is usually over-processed and will probably break because it is being scorched by a 350-degree hot curling iron rather than no perm. If the goal is to grow natural, then let the over-processed hair break. There is no need to try to save relaxed hair if your goal is to grow natural.

Assuming the hair is not over-processed and there is not a distinct line of demarcation from the new growth (see pg. 56), you may style the hair using a wet set or a pin-up style. Gel the edges flat and, if needed, tie the style in place for 15 minutes to make it neat. As more new growth comes in, a small roller wet set will blend the textured hair with the relaxed ends, or use a blow dryer comb nozzle to soften the new growth hair. For up styles, try a pompadour, French roll, hair tuck, sculptured up-do, flat twist or soft large braids.

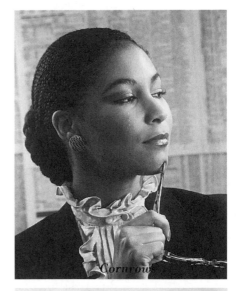

Cornrows

3. Hair extensions, braids & weaves

Braids, extensions and weaves are all considered transition styles. They keep your hair looking good while protecting it from daily wear and tear of combing and styling. It is a beautiful way to take the hair from the chemical stage to natural. Transition styles achieved using hair additions give you unlimited options to change the length, color and texture of your hair. As the hair is growing out with two different hair textures (new growth and chemical ends), it is less frustrating if the hair is covered and allowed to grow undisturbed. If the hair is weak, and the new growth is very different from the permed ends, a braid or extension does not add additional stress to the weak hair ends. Camouflaging the processed hair as new hair grows in makes the transition inconspicuous and beautiful at the same time.

Growing natural hair long is a gradual process; however, it is best to frequently clip off the

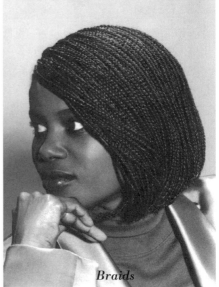

Braids

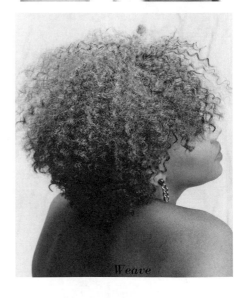

Weave

relaxed hair ends so that the hair will eventually be all one texture. Rather than be frustrated with hair that is becoming difficult to work with, let it rest. Curly hair grows fastest when it is combed and styled less often. Braids, twists and weaves give the hair that needed intermission from daily styling, hot curling, and "fixing." Unfortunately, many women use this style as a rest period, then return to chemical processing as soon as they see improvement and hair growth.

There are unlimited transition braids and extension styles. Braids and twist styles can be done without using hair additions. But if you are looking for a style that will last up to eight weeks, extensions are the answer. Individual braids with extension can be done in many different lengths and styles. This style offers lots of versatility and allows the scalp to breathe easily.

Individual braids are not recommended for the hurried person. On the average, this style can take up to eight hours or more. Because the style is labor intensive, you can expect to sit a while, even to remove the braids. Cornrow braid styles, on the other hand, are a delight because they do not take as long to do as individual braids and will give you a simple, stationary style. Some styles can take one hour, but the average cornrow style may take up to four hours. If the scalp is being treated with special products, cornrow braids may hinder easy access to the scalp; therefore, individual braids or a combination cornrow braids style would be best.

There is even a braid style for those of you who want the therapy of braids but do not want to see them. Yes, invisible braids styles like lace braids, interlock braids and hair weaves offer braids that are undetectable to the eye because the braids are hidden underneath the hair extension. They are usually done with human hair extension for easy styling. Lace braids are similar to individual braids, except the extension covers the individual braids.

For interlock braiding, the hair is cornrowed flat to the scalp and the extension comes out of the cornrow. With this extension style, you can cut the style shorter than your hair length without cutting into your hair.

The hair weave is wefts of hair sewn on to tracks of cornrows. The hair weave is especially good if you have thin and balding areas to cover or if you want a style that is contemporary and low maintenance. A full weave style can cover all of your hair, making it possible to try a different hair color or hair texture without the commitment. Some women want to cover their hair with a weave but want to maintain the same hair style as they were wearing before the weave. Yes, this is possible for the less daring.

4. Cover it up

For hair that is weak, fragile and in poor condition the previous options may not be possible. If you find yourself in this unfortunate position, don't panic or resort to a style that may further damage and weaken the hair. Let the hair and scalp slumber while new hair grows. Cover the hair and scalp with a wig, hat or fabric head wrap. The latter option will take some planning to be sure the head covering is stylish, coordinated, and comfortable. Head wraps should be fashionable but not tied tight.
Wigs can be cut and styled to suit your face shape; and hats should be lightweight to allow the scalp to breathe.

Growing out stages of chemically treated hair

Now that you know what styles are suitable for the transition, it is important that you are prepared and ready for the different stages your hair will go through as you are growing out the chemically treated hair.

There are some things we all take for granted, like knowing our hair texture and its characteristics. You might think that because you have lived with your hair all your life, you are familiar with how it feels, its curl pattern, and how it reacts to styling and handling. Realistically, many black women have straightened or altered their hair texture for so long that their natural hair is foreign and unfamiliar to them. It is not uncommon for women to go to the hair salon all of their adult life and never have to deal with doing their own hair. Like clockwork, their hair is chemically processed when they see a hint of natural curly, kinky hair growth. As quick as their natural hair grows in, it is soon forgotten because these women rush to the beauty parlor to get a chemical or press touch-up. And as much as some women say they want to grow the chemical out of their hair, fear of new growth sets in after the first several months. The kinky curl at the root is what these women have been taught to regard as "hard to comb and unsightly."

So many black women have straightened, relaxed and permed their hair for years, they have never had the opportunity to experience its true natural beauty. The average 30-year-old woman has been straightening her hair since childhood to adolescent; perhaps at least 20 years. And even though she may comb and groom her straight hair daily, she is not likely to experiment and explore what her natural hair texture can or cannot do.

I have found many women become depressed or apprehensive by the idea of growing the chemicals out of their hair. Women have complained that the new hair growth feels coarse and hard. This is usually an unfair analysis of natural hair that is compared to the straightened ends. I classify the first stage of new growth hair as the scab stage.

Hair that has been chemically processed for many years will grow out curlier and in some instances feel dry because of the long-time use of the caustic lye (relaxer) that has stripped the hair follicle of its natural oils and nutrients. Your hair goes through a healing process similar to a wound on the skin, which becomes supple again after the scab falls off. As the new hair growth lengthens, the follicle and scalp have a chance to be rejuvenated, heal and eventually replenish the natural sebum to the hair. The new hair will then begin to feel soft and pleasing. And of course, changing to hair care products that are formulated for curly hair will make a difference in how the hair looks and feels.

The beginning stage is the time to become re-acquainted with your hair and its natural characteristics. Expect the process to take some time and also expect a challenge as you will have to groom two opposing hair textures; the straight ends and the curly new growth. If you are not prepared for what kind of hair you have, the growing-out process can get more difficult as the new hair grows longer and thicker.

On an average, hair grows 6 inches per year. The chemically processed ends (if they do not break off) will need to be cut off gradually or all at once. If you decide to cut off all of the chemically processed hair and start all natural, then you will not go through these five transition stages of growing out the chemically treated hair. Up to a 20-month period, chemically treated hair goes through five recognizable growing out stages: *two months, six months, 10 months, 14 months, 20 months.*

Two months of new growth

The first stage is two months after the hair was chemically processed; the re-touch or "touch up" phase. There should be up to 1 inch of new-growth hair. At this stage the hair will not be very difficult to manage because of the small amount of new curly hair growth. It will only seem difficult, even impossible, to the "straight hair addict."

To flatten and smooth (not straighten) the curly, kinky edges, moisten the hairline area with wet hands, apply a very small amount of natural gel and tie the hair flat for at least 15 minutes with a cotton scarf. Another way to soften and smooth the new growth hair is to use the blow dryer comb nozzle to comb through and unwrinkle the natural hair so that it blends with the hair ends.

Six months of new growth

After six months you will notice three inches of curly hair at the scalp area. Blow dry the hair using a comb nozzle to loosen the natural curl enough to easily comb through the two hair textures. The objective is to try and blend the two textures. If the hair was over-processed and the ends are extremely straight, I recommended wearing braids or extensions to protect the ends from breaking.

Ten months

Bravo, you have come too far to turn back. You should have at least five inches of new growth hair visible. This hair will appear much thicker than the permed ends. Some of the straight ends may weaken and break off. This is not unusual and will happen until the relaxed ends are cut off. As the relaxed hair gets old, it also may tangle easily after a shampoo. The reason for tangling is that the imbrication on the cuticle layer of the relaxed ends are slightly open causing the hair strands to lock onto each other. If the hair ends mat, gently separate the matted hair with your fingers and apply a light liquid oil to the hair. The matting is an indication to begin cutting off the treated ends. Select a style that does not require the ends to show. Pin-up styles and extension styles will make the straight ends less noticeable. At this time, to start removing the straight ends clip one inch.

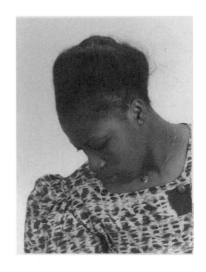

**Four months of new growth.
The sparse hairline
damaged from chemicals,
is growing back.**

Fourteen months of new growth

Almost there! Depending on the length your hair was when you started, one texture will be longer than the other. For example, if your hair was three inches or less when you started to grow out the chemical, you will have more natural hair than relaxed straight ends. If your hair was more than six inches long when you started to grow natural, you will still have quite a bit of chemical hair on the ends or half and half. The perm ends will appear thin. If it does not interfere with styling, trim off as much of the thin ends as possible. You should have at least seven inches of new hair.

20 months of new growth

You should have up to 10 inches of new hair. Because the natural hair is dominant, it may be very difficult to blend the two textures for styling, so rather than holding on, cut the straight ends down to the natural hair. Welcome to "all natural hair." The hair should feel soft, supple and have good elasticity and curl. And all coily, curly, kinky, natural hair has curl, but simply different size curls. Many natural styles are available to you now. Your selection of hair styles may include flat twist, up style braids, hanging braids and sculpted individual twist.

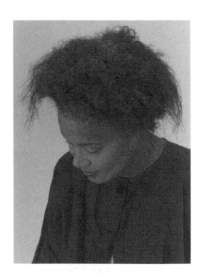

**Fourteen months of new growth
with 2 inches of relaxed ends
remaining.**

Experiment with styles that enhance your natural curl -- twist out, hand rolls, individual twist or just shape, style and wear your "freedom hair." And remember, to properly maintain and care for your freedom hair you must use products that are specially formulated for your natural hair texture. In addition, you can soften the hair and loosen the curly kink by using the dryer comb nozzle. This will make any hair texture easy to comb and comfortable to style. And since every person has very different hair texture, density, elasticity, and curliness, be careful not to compare your hair style results to a style you see on someone else's hair. Your hair texture will determine your individual style.

For women who will continue to use hair dyes and chemical cosmetics avoid using products with ingredients that are known carcinogens such as:

(all) Phenylenediamine	*Acid orange 87*
Acid violet 73	*Acid blue 168*
Solvent brown 44	*1,4-dioxane*
2,4 touenediamine	

Bibliography:

Palmer A, ET. AL. Respiratory disease prevalence in Cosmetologist and its relationship to aerosol sprays. Env. 1979: 19:136.

Osorio A, et. al. Investigation of lung cancer among female cosmetologist Journal of Occupational Medicine 1986;28:291

Spinelli JJ, et. al. Multiple Myeloma, Leukemia and Cancer of the Ovary in Cosmetologists and Hairdressers. Journal of Medicine 1983;25:871

Nethercott JR, et. al. Contact dermatitis in Hairdressers. Contact Dermatitis. 1986;14:73.

You can find these studies at the National Library of Medicine; Bethesda, Maryland.

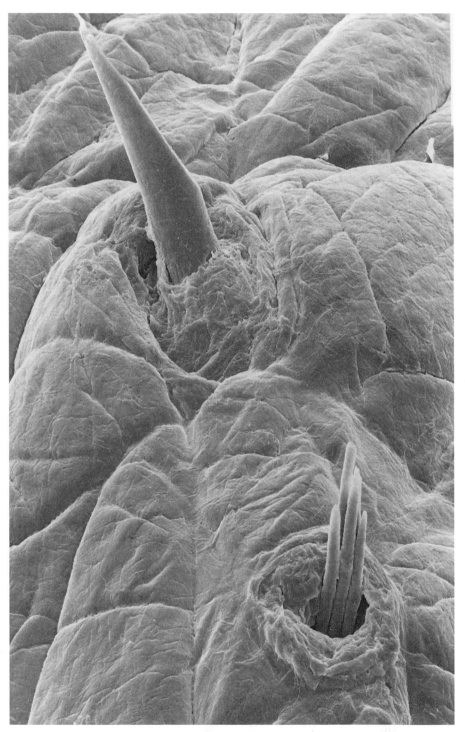

Magnified 1000 times, hair growing out of the hair follicle.

Photo Courtesy of Gillette Research Institute

A basic understanding of the human body and its functions is the best approach to learning about what makes your hair healthy and what can stimulate its growth. Healthy hair growth relies on a healthy body, pure circulating blood, and the life-giving properties from foods, and minerals.

Getting to Know

Your Hair

4

Your hair structure

Let's talk about hair, from the inside out. I believe it is important for you to be familiar with the structure of hair and some technical terms, as I will refer to these terms when I talk about hair care. If I were to say your cuticle layer is open, what does that mean to you?

There are six elements in the composition of hair: oxygen, hydrogen, carbon, nitrogen, sulfur, and phosphorus. To ensure average hair growth of at least 6" per year, your hair needs a constant supply of nourishment containing these elements. Wholesome, live foods that we eat are a vital source of these elements as well as the digestion of high quality proteins in the diet which begins the formation of hair. Hair is made up of a special protein, known as keratin. Important elements of protein include sulfur which gives the hair strength, and nitrogen, which is necessary for cellular growth and repair. The composition of the elements found in the hair vary based on a person's age, hair type, sex, racial origin, and hair color. The two parts to the hair are the shaft (above the scalp) and the root (below the scalp).

Above the scalp.........hair shaft
The hair shaft has three layers
1. The outer layer is the *cuticle*;
2. The middle layer is the *cortex*;
3. The innermost layer is the *medulla.*

The hair **cuticle** is the outer protective layer. It has overlapping layers (imbrications) similar to fish scales. These imbrications overlap away from the scalp. Let me give you an example of why this is important.

If you rub fish scales in the direction they are pointing they feel smooth, as the translucent scales protect the inner flesh. Rub the scales in the opposite direction and the open scales will feel rough, and expose the inner flesh to whatever can penetrate it. Imagine the first layer (cuticle) of hair like this. If the cuticle is healthy, the hair will feel smooth and will not tangle easily. Damaged hair will have cuticles that are open, missing and poorly arranged, as a fish left with its scales rubbed backward.

In some cases you want the cuticles to open. For instance, during a deep-heat condition treatment, the heat opens the cuticle allowing the conditioner to penetrate to the second layer, and then the cool rinse will close the healthy cuticle layer back. The risk of harsh chemical applications is that the chemical can destroy some of the cuticle (protective) layer, exposing the hairs inner layers (cortex and medulla) and making it vulnerable to damage.

The **cortex** is the second (strength) layer where the pigment granules (natural hair color) and structural bonds are found. So if you lighten your hair color, the process involves going into this second layer and removing the natural pigment from the granules. The structural bonds determine the genetic shape and form of the hair (wavy, curly, straight). The shape can be re-arranged temporarily by physically styling the hair or permanently by chemically manipulating the bonds.

The **medulla** layer is evidently not one of the more important layers since some hair types lack it. It is the most inner layer made of soft keratin. Thick hair will always have a medulla, layer; thin, fine hair may not.

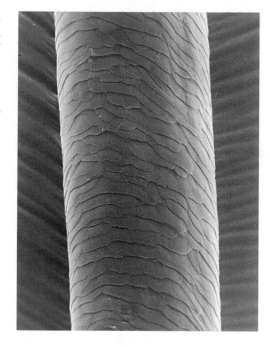

A strand of healthy hair magnified 1000 times. The cuticle is like a shield.

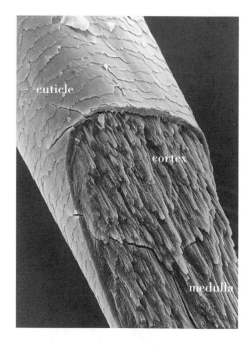

A cross-section of hair showing the three layers; cuticle, cortex and medulla

Below the scalp..........hair root

The hair root is that part of the hair hidden below the scalp. It consists of a *follicle, glands , papilla, hair bulb, and blood vessels.*

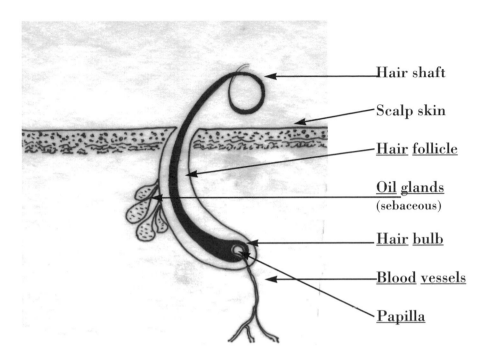

Hair shaft

Scalp skin

Hair follicle

Oil glands
(sebaceous)

Hair bulb

Blood vessels

Papilla

Follicle -- A pocket that holds the hair root and determines the shape of the hair.

Oil (Sebaceous) Glands -- Each hair strand has gland sacs attached to the wall of the follicle. The glands produce sebum (oil), which lubricates the hair for sheen and keeps the hair moist and supple.

Papilla -- At the very bottom of the hair follicle is a part of the skin that is in contact with the blood vessels. The hair receives a rich blood and nerve supply that contributes to the hairs growth through the papilla. If the papilla deteriorates, the hair will never grow.

Hair bulb -- the end part of the hair root which covers the papilla.

Blood vessels -- small veins to transport the nutrients from the blood to the hair papilla.

Hair Characteristics

Texture is how hair feels and looks curly, straight, soft, coarse, wiry, silky, cottony, thick or fine. It is not unusual to find several different hair textures on one head. For instance, the hair may be fine with a loose curl in the nape area and thick with a small curl in the crown.

Density is the amount of hair per square inch of the scalp. One can have dense hair whether the hair type is thick or fine. In this sense, dense is synonymous with plentiful, so hair can be fine and still be dense.

Diameter is the circular thickness of a strand of hair. If the hair strand is thin, the diameter is considered small or referred to as fine. The hair strand that is thick has a bigger diameter. This can be compared to feeling different weights of thread, some are very fine while others, like carpet thread, are thick.

Elasticity gives hair its strength. It is the ability of the hair to be stretched and return to its original length without breaking. Hair that has good elasticity will not break when you stretch it. Hair that has poor elasticity will break easily when stretched, pulled or even styled.

Porosity is the hair strands ability to absorb moisture and water. Good porosity is recognized by hair that wets easily and consistently. If the hair does not wet easily, it is resistant to water and has poor porosity. Hair that wets quickly and absorbs too much water is over-porous. Tinted, bleached and chemically over-processed hair is typically over-porous.

Characteristics of curly hair types

African-American people, especially, have hair textures that range from fine to thick and straight to coily. Because curly and coily hair texture is seldom discussed in any hair styling and care books, my concentration will be on these textures of hair. In this section we will learn some general African-American hair characteristics like curl size, frizz, shrinkage, light absorption, and swelling. The one distinct difference in many African-American hair textures is the size of the curls. I will categorize three general size curls I have found in the many clients who have come to my natural hair salon.

If you were to examine your curl (coil) size throughout your hair, you will find it is larger in some areas where the hair may appear wavy long, while in other areas the curl is smaller, causing the hair to shrink more. The hair line or edges are usually finer, softer and shorter than the interior hair. The crown in many cases is thickest if the hair is healthy. Identifying the curls and textures of your hair will help you choose the correct styles that enhance your hairs characteristics.

Once you are familiar with your hair characteristics, it is especially important to use products that are formulated for your hair type. Using the wrong shampoo, condition-er or other hair products can change the way your hair may naturally curl, swell, shrink, or feel; giving a false appearance to your hair's true characteristics. Knowing this, helps you to recognize when your hair does not feel or look normal. It gives you the knowledge to judge if what you have done to your hair is good for it.

Through examination of the hair strands from hundreds of heads, I have discovered that African-American hair is typically *wavy, curly or coily*. The wavy hair type is mostly uniform curves and bends in hair that is a combination of straight and curly. Curly hair is like wavy hair but with a smaller size curl and coil combination. The coily, crinkly hair is more common and prevalent for African-Americans. Each hair strand has uneven curves, bends and coils. As a group, the hair strands look like a mass of differently directed curls but upon close examination, the curls are not consistent throughout the hair strand. Pull a strand of hair from your head while the hair is wet and look at the irregular curls and bends. What makes this hair type so special and unique is that no two strands of hair are the same.

General curl (bend) sizes.

1. **Wavy curl has a loose bend curl about 1/2"-1," giving the hair a uniform wave and smooth appearance.**

2. **Curly hair has a medium size curl that measures about 1/8 - 1/4".**
(see the two examples in the illustration)

3. **Coily hair is recognized by a tight or very small curl size measuring 1/8" or smaller.**

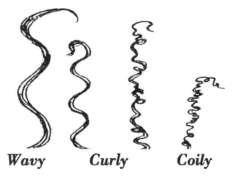

Wavy   Curly   Coily

What is the natural curl size in your hair?
Here are two (2) simple steps to identify your natural curl size.

1.) To find the curl size of your hair, wet your hair thoroughly then saturate it with hair conditioner to examine the curl pattern that forms in the hair. The hair closest to the scalp will give a good indication of your hair's curl pattern.

2.) **Rinse the hair thoroughly. Pluck out a strand of hair from the crown and tape each end to a piece of blank paper (do not stretch). Place a ruler along the hair to measure the distance of each bend and examine the curl/crinkle size. If the formation of the hair is irregular and not uniform, find the dominant bends (curl) in the hair strand and this will give you a good indication of the size curl throughout your hair. Keep in mind hair has different textures throughout the head, so measure hairs from different areas of the head.**

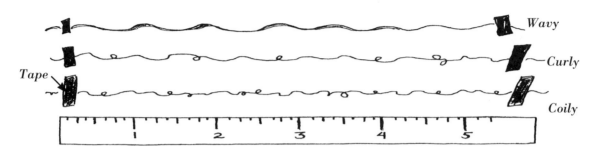

Use the ruler to measure the natural curl size in your hair. Tape the two ends (do not stretch the hair strand). Measure the distance of each bend throughout the hair.

The degree of crinkle and curliness is based on the curl size. In some hair textures, the curl is very defined and uniform and you can easily see curls in the hair when it is moist. In other hair textures, the curl is sporadic throughout the hair strand. This is what makes hair frizzy and kinky looking. Because hair strands are irregular and different, it may take practice to accurately classify your natural curl size. Examine the hair for curl formation and match it to the general curl size.

How does your natural hair feel?

Cottony, spongy, heavy, wiry, or wispy? African-American hair is so unique it is only fair to analyze it in three different stages; wet, naturally dry, and blown dry smooth.

Cottony hair, a fine texture with 50 percent or more shrinkage, actually feels soft and airy like cotton. Cotton soft hair is most affected by humidity and happiest "au natural."

Spongy hair, medium to thick texture with 65 percent or more shrinkage, feels firm and cushiony to the touch. It usually has a medium to small tight crinkle. When wet, the hair is very dense.

Heavy hair texture has a large diameter and a deep strong curl. This hair is typically recognized as if it is a mixture of Native American or Asian hair type with African hair. It may shrink about 40 percent or less.

Wiry hair has a glossy finish and is not very pliable. The hair diameter is usually large and the crinkle is loose. Although this hair type may have a thick diameter, it is often not dense at the crown and is mixed with non-wiry hair. The shrinkage will vary because the wiry hair does not shrink much but the other hair does.

Wispy hair is fine, thin, very lightweight and fly away. This texture hair will feel static if the correct shampoo is not used. The shrinkage depends on how curly the wispy hair is.

Hair Shrinkage

There are some things you can expect African American hair textures to do -- curl, swell, frizz and shrink. Because there is a strong resilient curl and crinkle, certain climate conditions may encourage the hair to do any of these things. Any kind of moisture will make the hair shrink and frizz. Heat and humidity will cause the hair to swell and expand, more noticeably for curly hair. Heat makes hair swell and puff; cold makes it contract and feel inflexible. The hair strands inconsistent crinkle and curl is what makes natural hair appear frizzy. Frizz is simply a mass of curls and crinkles that give the hair a wrinkle effect.

Your hair's weight and curl size determine how much it will coil and shrink. Thin hair with small curls shrinks more than heavy hair with large curls. The shrinkage is judged by measuring the difference in the length of wet hair compared to when it is blown dry smooth or stretched out. If you were to blow dry the hair smooth or stretch a piece of wet hair outward, you would be able to see its entire length. For example, wet natural hair may appear to be five inches long but once the hair is blown smooth, it is 12" long. Blown dry smooth is like uncoiling the natural hair; except the hair still maintains some texture and crinkle. How much does your hair draw up and recoil when it is moistened or wet?

Once you know the curl pattern and common characteristics of your hair, choosing styles that are enhanced by wrinkles, puffiness, or frizz will be the most care-free. When you try to fight and combat these natural tendencies you can ruin your hair. Of course there are chemically processed styles that can prevent the hair from undergoing these natural changes. However, the after effects should cause concern. If natural hair is your aim, the idea is not to fight or change the hairs natural beauty, but to choose a style that compliments the crinkle texture and makes the natural curl radiant and more uniform. In addition, certain temporary styling techniques can re-shape the natural curl. By using the twist technique, a roller set or sculpted styles, you can manage and define the hairs true beauty. The styles that are achieved using the natural curl are less likely to shrink or swell because the hair is at that stage already. What a relief.

CURL SIZE	SHRINKAGE	FULL LENGTH
Large curl	15 - 30 percent shrinkage	1/4 its full length.
Medium curl	35 - 50 percent shrinkage	1/2 full length.
Small curl	75 or + percent shrinkage	3/4 full length.

Here are two ways to test your hair's shrinkage:

On average, African-American hair will shrink between 20 to 85 percent. The greater the shrinkage, the tighter and shorter the hair is when wet. You can measure your hair's shrinkage on blow dried hair or stretch the hair while it is wet.

1. Blow dry smooth

a) After shampooing, comb out and make small sections.
b) Blow dry each section smooth.
c) Compare the wet hair to the blown dry hair in order to determine an estimated percentage of shrinkage.

2. Stretch the hair

(If you don't blow dry the hair, the other way is to stretch the hair out.)
a) After wetting the hair, grasp the ends of a small section and stretch the hair out to its full length.
b) Compare the length of the wet hair and stretched hair.

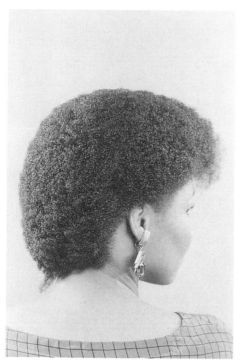
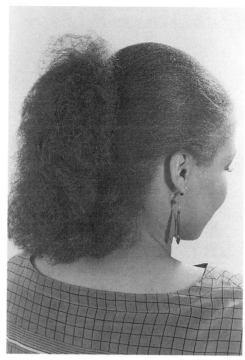

Blow dry smooth
This clients hair (left) shrinks about 75 percent of its full length.
The hair was blow dried (right) to compare the shrinkage.

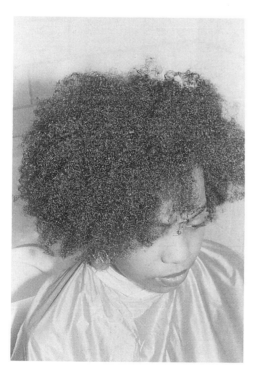
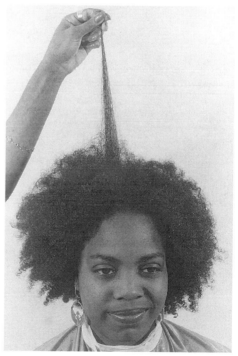

Stretch the hair
If you don't want to blow dry the hair, stretch the hair to see it's full length.

Selecting the right products

Recognizing your hair condition is the key to selecting the right products in order to personalize your hair care. First identify your hair type and condition.

Normal hair can be recognized as being healthy, not too oily nor too dry, has good elasticity, porosity, natural shine and grows well.

Dry hair feels coarse, brittle and stiff. It is not getting enough oils and moisture. An under-active oil gland may be the cause for this hair condition. Another common misconception is that curly, kinky hair is dry. This misjudgment is usually based on one of two things, (1) dark color curly hair does not reflect light, therefore, it may appear to lack luster and sheen, (2) curly hair also is often treated with products designed for straight hair that have de-greasing agents that will strip all the natural oils from the hair, making it feel dry. Shampoos that have harsh detergents also will make the hair look ashy and dry. Another culprit is the chemicals in municipal water systems. For example, the chlorine in treated water may remove pigment and cause the hair to look dull.

Oily hair feels greasy and sticky as if it has a film on it. An overactive sebaceous gland produces too much oil for the hair or a build-up of greasy products. With this hair condition the excess oil can make the hair difficult to style, and odorous, if the oil build-up is not frequently shampooed off the scalp.

Dry scalp is a tight scalp that has small fine flakes of dandruff or no dandruff but an ashy appearance. The scalp is dehydrated, lacking the natural protective oil produced by the sebaceous gland that keeps the scalp supple and moist.

Oily scalp has large flaking dandruff. The sebaceous gland is producing oil but the scalp cannot rid itself fast enough of the new cell layers that the oil adheres to. Oily scalp will also make the face oily and prone to acne. Coating an oily type scalp problem with grease and heavy pomades only aggravates the condition.

Itchy scalp occurs if old cells accumulate faster than they are eliminated. This will cause a build-up of oil and dead cells, creating a flaking and itchy scalp condition. Other factors that can cause the scalp to itch are infrequent shampoos, insufficient rinsing, nervous disorder, synthetic extensions, and allergic reaction to cosmetics and chemicals in tap water.

Dandruff does not always mean the scalp is dry. The scalp can be oily or can become irritated from shampoo detergents, not rinsing thoroughly, and too frequent shampooing which strips away the skins natural oils. In some cases, you may have a skin disorder such as seborrhea or psoriasis; if so, contact a scalp specialist or dermatologist.

Always consult your hair care stylist about your hair type, its condition and selecting the right hair care and styling products. The most common mistake people make in hair care is using the wrong products. For example, shampoos formulated for blonde silky hair, is of no benefit to dark curly tresses. Until you find the best products for your hair texture you will never experience or come to appreciate your hair's true beauty. Even today, there are too few good products made for curly, kinky, crinkly hair. Many product manufacturers, including African-American companies, make their products for straight or straightened hair textures. They advertise showing the natural hair as if it is a mess; damaged or untouched by beauty, until you use their shampoo, promising to make your hair straight and manageable. Look for products that celebrate the beauty and true essence of your natural hair. It is contradictory to promote a product for black hair and portray the black woman with naturally crinkly hair as bad and ugly, and straight hair as the good and ultimate goal. Avoid these products on mere principle alone and leave them for women who desire or have that kind of hair.

The difference between straight and curly, crinkly hair types is significant. Straight hair types are usually more likely to be oily, and the shampoo and conditioner are formulated to remove these oils from the hair shaft so the hair is not weighted down and stringy. De-greasing products are intended to give more body and fluff to Caucasian hair by eliminating the oil. On the other hand, the black woman's hair has natural body and fluff and loves oils. This hair type needs to retain as much of its natural oil (sebum) as possible. Because of the many bends and curves in curly hair, the natural oil does not distribute evenly on the hair shaft, so using products that are rich in natural oil similar to the body's sebum is a way of helping nature do its job. Products formulated for curly, kinky hair have more emollients, fatty acids and are not de-greasing. Since the shampoo is non de-greasing, it is not necessary to replace your hair oils after shampooing. If the product does not strip the hair and has natural oils in the formulation, it is good for curly, crinkly hair.

How do you know if it is formulated for your hair? Don't be fooled by the red, black and green colors, nor the black women's faces on the product labels. This is often a marketing tool where the image is made for you but the product is not. Unfortunately, the very best natural products formulated for African-American hair are made by small, little known companies where the chemists or "cosmetic chefs" experiment on their own hair and are truly dedicated to a wholesome product. Learn to read labels and distinguish between ingredients that curly hair likes and ingredients you should avoid.

Also be mindful that there are different qualities and quantities of substances used in the many shampoos, conditioners, gels and oils. In other words, two different shampoo products may have similar ingredients; however the amount used, the quality and where the ingredient comes from can make the two products distinctly different. To get an idea of how much of an ingredient is in a cosmetic, remember that the ingredients are listed in the order of most quantity to least. For example, if water is the first ingredient and herbal extract is the last ingredient, the product has mostly water in its formulation.

The advantage to natural hair care is that fewer products are needed for maintaining the hair. Natural hair care is simple and basic. Shampoo, conditioner, hair oil, and a natural styling gel are all you need. There is no need for the daily use of heavy grease, mousse, spritz, or hard hair sprays. And if the label has too many ingredients that you do not recognize or can't pronounce, it would be safe to avoid this product until you know the substances.

Some common natural ingredients are cocamide, shea butter, jojoba, citric acid, aloe vera, royal jelly, vitamin E, vegetable glycerin, plant based essential fatty acids, flower, plant and seed extracts and oils, lecithin, sea plants and minerals.

A Good Shampoo

Shampoos are formulated to cleanse the hair and scalp without adversely affecting them. In other words you may have a shampoo that deep cleanses the hair but may be harsh on the scalp, causing it to irritate and become dry. Or you may use a shampoo that is effective for dandruff, but it makes the hair feel hard and look dull. The objective is to find a product that is gentle and nourishing to both the hair and skin. There is no one shampoo that suits every hair type and hair need, so finding the best shampoo for your hair may take some experimentation. Asking someone who has similar hair, or through the process of elimination are good starts. There is no easier method to selecting the right shampoo other than trying several kinds and finding the one that works best for you. There are, however, some basic things that can help you to eliminate certain products. If you can narrow down your choices, the process will not take forever nor be compromised. For example, shampoo that is designed to make straight hair silky is not for curly, kinky hair, and shampoo for curly hair will make straight hair flat and heavy. More often, chemically straightened hair needs some oil where naturally straight hair does not.

As your hairs condition and needs change with the seasons and climate, you may have to alternate shampoo brands. A shampoo that may be perfect in the summer may not be as effective during the winter months. This is not always the case, but some cities and states have very different climates creating special hair needs. Another concern is whether your tap water is hard or soft and what chemicals are used to treat it. The quality of water will make a difference in how the shampoo will lather or effect dryness of the scalp. However, if you find the right product for your hair type, it can serve you well for a lifetime.

The best shampoo is one that keeps the scalp moist and supple while leaving the hair soft and easy to comb. Look for shampoos that have naturally derived ingredients. The fewer ingredients in the product the better. Although color and fragrance help trigger many women to buy products, they have no health benefit. Look for naturally derived fragrances and colorants such as annato, black walnut, sage, red clover and other vegetable, root and herbs sources instead of artificial ingredients. Some natural cosmetics will even have a minimal amount of preservative or artificial substances. All products, even the natural ones, need a preservative to prevent bacterial growth and contaminant's from repeatedly opening and closing the bottle. The preservative also gives the cosmetic product shelf life, to prevent spoilage and separation. Although chemical preservatives are usually the least expensive and are very effective, there are some naturally derived preservatives like citrus and menthol. Naturally derived preservatives, however, may increase the cost of the product. The only "all natural" cosmetic is one that you make at home. If you wish to have a pure, totally natural cosmetic, you will have to make your own in small quantities.

Common ingredients found in shampoos are:

Potassium Cocoate - A highly saturated fat derived from coconut kernels (coconut oil) for lathering. May be irritating to skin.

Lauramide DEA - The principal fatty acid of coconut oil used as a softener and foaming agent.

Cocamidoproply Betaine - same as coconut oil.

Glycol Stearate - A mixture of glycerin and alcohol used as a humectant. Some glycols may be harmful in large concentrations.

Methyparaben - A widely used preservative that has anti-microbial activity; can cause allergic reactions.

Sodium chloride - Same as common table salt, used as an astringent.

Disodiumlauryl sulfosuccinate - Wetting agent used where mildness is important.

Lauryl sulfate - derived from laurel alcohol, which is produced from coconut oil and used for its foaming properties.

Ammonium lauryl sulfate - a mild acidic surfactant that is the ammonium salt that comes from coconut alcohol. May cause curly hair to become dry.

Sodium lauryl sulfate -Less drying than Ammonium; wetting agent, cleansing agent. May cause dryness because of its degreasing ability.

Dandruff Shampoos

A number of commercial dandruff shampoos work on mild cases of dry flaking scalp. For excessive dandruff, psoriasis, or seborrhea, use a natural shampoo that is gentle enough to use frequently. To prevent the hair from becoming dry, use the dandruff shampoo in moderation, applying to the scalp only, and use a regular shampoo to clean the hair shaft. A strong tea rinse made from burdock root, rosemary and/or thyme can be used as a natural remedy for dandruff.

Common ingredients found in dandruff shampoos are :

Zinc pyrithione - An anti-dandruff ingredient; reportedly damaging to the nerves.
Sulfur - A mild antiseptic, this comes from the earth's crust (brimstone). It may
    cause irritation to the skin.
Tars - Obtained by the distillation of wood, coal and peat; this antiseptic can cause
    skin irritations or allergic reactions.
Salicylic acid - An antiseptic used for anti-itch, it absorbs through the skin; large
    amounts cause skin rashes, stomach pain an acidosis.
Resorcinol - This preservative, anti-itch and anti-fungal agent can cause irritation
    to the mucus membranes and skin.

Good Hair Conditioner

Hair conditioners are like lotion to the hair. Many conditioners will have humectants to help maintain moisture in the hair, and finishing agents that leave a coating on the hair to make it feel softer. Now that women are using strong chemical cosmetics and heat styling tools, the need for conditioning and restoring the hair shaft has become greater. This does not mean hair conditioners can repair damaged hair. Conditioners were made to do what sebum oil does naturally -- provide a protective lubricant to the hair to make the scalp supple and the hair pliable. Conditioners with natural oils will give luster to the hair shaft, making it appear glossy. A good conditioner should disappear when hands are rubbed together.

Cream rinse or leave-in hair conditioners are recommended after each shampoo to maintain moisture, and give lubrication and luster to the hair. A cream rinse should be used regularly but if the hair is extremely damaged, there is not much a hair conditioner can do to restore good health. Therefore, use the conditioner as a maintenance treatment rather than as an emergency repair product.

Cream Rinse Conditioner is a finishing product to coat the hair shaft, leaving a film that makes the hair moist and supple. The conditioner is applied to the scalp and hair after the shampoo. Most cream rinse conditioners are left on the hair for several minutes and then rinsed off with cool water. Be sure to follow the manufacturer's directions on all products. Some cream rinse conditioners may build up a residue on the hair.

Leave-In Conditioner is applied to the hair after a shampoo and left on for added protection from styling and handling. They usually contain substances that help to bring moisture to the hair. This type of conditioner is best suited for hair that needs extra moisture and will be styled naturally or with heat. <u>Avoid using too much leave-in conditioner</u> because it will make the hair look ashy, feel sticky, lay flat, and difficult to style.

Deep Conditioner is a treatment that penetrates the hair's cuticle layer. It is called deep conditioner because it is enhanced by body, steam or electric heat. The heat dilates the cuticle layer of the hair strand, causing the rich conditioner to enter into the inner layers of the hair.

Some ingredients found in hair conditioners are:

Lanolin - Derived from the oil glands of a sheep, lanolin is intended to help the skin absorb and hold water.

Mineral oil - Liquid petroleum, non-toxic, mineral oil remains on the skin surface rather than absorbing into the skin.

Spermaceti - An emollient used to improve gloss, spermaceti is wax drawn from the head of the sperm whale.

Monostearate- A naturally fatty acid found in butter and tallow, monostearate gives the pearly color to products.

Alcohol - Made from the fermentation of carbohydrates, alcohol is a fat solvent that can cause dryness to the hair and scalp.

Sterols - This is a solid complex alcohol that comes from animals and plants.

Good Hair Oil

Oil is used today by African-Americans very much like it was in Ancient Africa. Natural oils derived from plants and flowers, occasionally animals (lanolin from oil glands of sheep), are used for medicinal, curative and cosmetic purpose. In some cases, people apply oil to the hair and scalp from habit rather than necessity. If the scalp is cleansed frequently, the oil glands are normal, and the hair products used have sufficient nutrient oils, then daily oiling of the hair and scalp is not needed. However if you feel you need extra sheen on the hair, and to keep moisture on the scalp, light natural oils should be used.

When the scalp does not produce a sufficient amount of sebum on the hair shaft, hair oils can be used to supplement this deficiency. Liquid natural oils are recommended over heavy grease and synthetic oils (petroleum and mineral oil) because of their penetrating quality. Synthetic oils do not absorb into the skin easily, they simply coat the skins surface. If synthetic oils are used regularly and not cleansed from the scalp thoroughly, they can build up on the skin and create blockage in the hair follicle, suffocating hair growth. Synthetic oils are used in many products because these oils are less costly, the supply is unlimited and they do not go rancid like natural oils. When purchasing natural oils, buy in small quantities.

Some naturally derived oils may be too concentrated to apply directly to the skin; therefore a base oil is used in hair oil combinations. Some base oils are *olive, castor, almond, coconut, jojoba, glycerin, soybean and safflower.*

Jojoba oil, used for centuries by Native Americans, is extracted from the seeds of the Simondsia Chinensis desert shrub. This oil is very similar to human sebum. It removes embedded sebum from the hair follicle and makes the scalp less acidic. Most plant, flower, and fruit oils have some unique therapeutic and nutrient properties.

Hair Gel, and Holding Hair Spray

While hair gels can come in many forms, the intended use is for molding, sculpting and holding the hair in place. Heavy gels are for a firm hold and lacquer effect and light gels keep hair frizz and swelling to a minimum. Some of the ingredients found in gels: Aloe Vera, marshmallow root, gum arabic blend, carbomer 940, copolymer, and flax seed.

As mentioned earlier, ingredients in holding sprays cause nerve, kidney and liver damage. Aerosol hair sprays are to be used sparingly, and always outdoors or in well-ventilated rooms. If you should use hair spray once a year, that may be too much. Many women and cosmetologists do not realize how dangerous and toxic aerosol hair spray can be. One of the ingredients in hair sprays, methylene chloride, is banned from use as an ingredient in cosmetics. It is a narcotic and highly toxic. Natural gums such as tragacanth and gum arabic are used in hair sprays; however, they can cause allergic reactions, gastrointestinal distress and asthma.

Safe Natural Hair Color

The most natural woman may feel a need to enhance her hair color, cover gray hair, add color to brighten dull faded hair, or completely change the natural hair color. Safe vegetable hair colors are available that coat the hair shaft rather than open the cuticle layer and interfere with the hairs natural pigment. The natural hair color process can only give color, it can not take it away; so to naturally lighten your dark hair color would not be possible. To lighten the hair would involve removing the color pigment (within the second layer of the hair), then depositing another color to the bleached pigment. The advantage of natural derived and plant base hair colors is that they are mild and should not damage the hair structure. Some hair colors will stain the hair shaft to leave a permanent lasting hair color while others are so mild that the color is simply a shade that fades with shampooing. To be sure to have a consistent color, it is best to have it done by a hair color specialist. Some natural choices are vegetable colorants, color rinses, color shampoo and stick color.

Vegetable color is a powder of dried herbs, and roots mixed with water into a paste to color the hair. This type of color gives the most intense long-lasting color

Color rinses are made from strong tea of the dried herbs and water. The rinse is poured through the hair to remain until the next shampoo.

Color shampoos are a combination of herbal colorant and shampoo. This is used to enhance faded and dull hair color.

Stick colors are a color wax stick used to touch up the growth of new hair between color treatments.

Natural colors are derived from plant roots, leaves, flowers, berries, fruit and vegetable skins. Some of the herbs commonly used to color hair are sage, indigo, black walnut, hollyhock, alkanet, annato and henna. The henna hair color has a tendency to make the hair feel dry and coarse. I have found, if you add olive oil or an egg yolk, this will soften the mixture and prevent drying the hair. Also deep condition the hair after the color process.

Until more research and experimentation are done using herbal hair colors, the one disadvantage is that the color range for natural coloring is limited. Chemical hair colorants offer a wider range of color and shades. Some women may choose to use semi-permanent hair color because of the wide range of colors. If so, deep conditioning treatments and natural styling is recommended as a gentle means of handling the fragile hair. This may help to prevent dryness and breakage. Always try to select a hair color that is one shade different from your natural color so that the new growth will not be as noticeable as the hair grows out. Also, this will allow you to go a longer period between color touch-ups. There is nothing worse than seeing a woman with white roots and black dyed ends or vice-a-versa.

If your beautician mixes hair color with hydrogen peroxide, or a "booster," you are not receiving a natural color. The peroxide penetrates the cuticle so that the color can stain the cortex layer. Chemical hair color (aniline tints, metallic dyes) do not change the basic structure of the hair texture; however the process can weaken the hair shaft because it affects the inner layer of the hair. The most damaging hair color process uses ammonia, hydrogen peroxide, and bleach lightener on the hair. This can cause the hair to feel dry, and brittle causing it to break. The ammonia used in the hydrogen peroxide will strip the hair of its natural oils in the cuticle, making the hair dry like straw. Compounding the damage, many women will relax their hair then use chemical hair color, too. Chemically straightening and coloring the hair is a sure way to ruin it. This double process is exposing the hair to two chemicals, increasing the risk of permanently damaging the cuticle protective layer, making the middle cortex layer vulnerable to the simplest of hair styling (i.e. rollers, heat apparatus and combing). Again if you should have the double process chemical treatment, always have it done by a licensed cosmetologist who specializes in this service.

To keep naturally grey hair from yellowing

Maintaining your naturally gray and white hairs true color is the key to graying beautifully. As hair loses its pigment, dark hair is replaced with white hair. In contrast to the dark hair the white gives the illusion of gray color. However, hair does not gray, it actually whitens. As with anything white, there is a tendency for it to get dingy, yellowed and discolored. There is nothing worse than dingy, discolored white hair; it makes the hair look dirty and aged. I have found that prevention is the first defense and maintenance is a backup. Here are some reasons why white hair will dull and yellow.

Infrequent shampooing. Daily styling products, scalp perspiration and pollutants in the air creates a build-up on the hair if it is not regularly shampooed. These oils and dirt stain the white hair.

Using the wrong products. Gels, gummy hair sprays, and colored shampoos can cause discoloring. White hair is a special hair; although it is resistant and not as porous as darker hair, using hair products that have lifting substances and color ingredients can stain your precious white strands.

Scorching the hair. Repeatedly pressing or hot curling grey hair will cause it to become yellow, brown and sometimes brittle. There is not much you can do to reverse the browning of burned scorched hair. Always test on a white towel and regulate the heat of hot curling irons and pressing combs before touching the hair. To prevent this accident from happening, select styles that do not require direct heat.

In some cases the yellowed hair can be treated to bring back the whiteness. It is best to consult a professional who is familiar with color balancing. Slight discolorations can be corrected with a bluing rinse. A series of special treatments are needed for more intense discoloration.

Other tips for safe and healthy hair coloring are:

1. *Avoid all products with **Phenylenediamine;** most dark colors will have this substance.*
2. *Have your color specialist use techniques like painting, frosting and streaking color tones onto the hair. This process does not apply the color directly onto the scalp.*
3. *Use color to highlight grey rather than cover it completely. Many natural colors do not give 100% coverage on white, however a 40% coverage will give warm tones.*

Herbal Hair Color Chart

For Dark Hair	Purple Sage (to darken gray hair), black walnut shell, indigo elderberries
For Light Hair	Yarrow, camomile, hollyhock (to brighten)
For Gray Hair	Betony (to enhance and brighten), Hollyhock (purplish blue flowers)
For Red Hair	Saffron, sassafras root, red clover (enhances color)

(The herbal rinses enhance your hair color; they do not change it)

Hair Problems

While most women will come to the hair salon feeling there is a problem with their hair, many can be remedied. A greater percentage of hair problems are reversible because they are physical problems with the hair shaft, but the smaller and more alarming are the hair problems that are systemic (from internal dis-ease). Physically created hair problems can be caused by using the wrong hair products, poor hygiene, residue build-up from excessive finishing sprays, and gels, or scorching the hair with a hot styling apparatus. Even damage to the hair shaft from excessive chemical hair treatments can be reversed. The most common problems encountered in the hair salon, like breaking, dullness, dryness and shedding, can be restored with good hygiene, deep penetrating scalp and hair treatments, and protective styling.

Systemic hair problems, on the other hand, are either early or advanced signs of an acute illness, vitamin deficiency or other serious health problem. Poor hair and scalp condition is one of the external indicators to tell that something is not functioning well within the body. Unfortunately, women do not heed to the early warning signs the body will give via the hair. The most challenging part of hair care for the hair care specialist is to try and obtain enough information from the client to be able to offer help. This is not always easy because many women are not "in tune" to their bodies or cognizant of their daily habits. Even though each client is treated individually with her unique circumstance, it is still like trying to piece together a puzzle. The bits and pieces you can get the client to remember and be honest about is the vital information that can give answers to that client's particular hair problem. If she has never viewed her hair as an intricate part of the body, important details are overlooked and often dismissed. Usually women are looking for a band-aid treatment that will make the hair pretty, out of sight-out of mind, but they never attempt to get to the root of the problem.

I have had clients come to the salon with male pattern baldness and act as if this is normal. They would say it runs in their family. And when I would question them whether they are on medication, or have diabetes, fibroids, a hysterectomy, high blood pressure, syphilis, thyroid problems or poor blood circulation, the response is often a non-chalant "no I don't have any of these problems, I'm perfectly healthy." A woman who is losing her hair is not perfectly healthy. This should be of more concern than covering the head with a pretty hair style. Granted, I know if a woman looks good she will feel good; however, obvious abnormal hair problems can be an early warning sign to a serious health problem.

One of my clients had been wearing a hair weave for several years, but her hair seemed to be getting shorter and thinner at the temple and hairline. This was unusual because the braided hair weave typically promotes hair growth. Each time she came to the salon I would question her to see if she was doing something to the hair or if she was experiencing any changes in her health. On each successive visit she started to open up and remember what she considered changes in her health that she had earlier dismissed as working too hard and thought that it would pass. She began to tell me the bits and pieces; she had missed her menstrual cycle for five months, experienced hand shakes, fatigue and had a frightening dizzy spell. It turned out that she had a hyperactive thyroid and a large growing fibroid in her uterus. These two health problems were causing a change in her hair. Unfortunately, women will go to the beauty salon before they will go to the doctor; so if the salon is a safe place to encourage clients to monitor their well being and seek medical help as needed, the stylist must pay attention to what the hair is revealing.

In addition to visually analyzing the hair shaft, the hair can be used to accurately assess toxic concentrations of minerals in the body. This is called a "hair analysis." It is a non invasive process that can determine exposure to toxic elements like lead, mercury and cadmium. A small clipping of natural hair is removed from the nape or pubic area and then a reading is done to determine the intracellular concentration of these substances. The hair analysis has been proven to be a more reliable test for mineral substances than urine and serum specimens. This method is helpful to prescribe nutritional supplements and treatment for a patient who may have a chemical imbalance or toxic chemical storage in the body. A hair analysis should be done by a health practitioner or trichologist (hair specialist).

Some causes for hair loss

Hair loss can be permanent or temporary and is characterized by thinning, shedding and the absence of hair on the head. Permanent hair loss is irreversible and cannot be changed. This form of hair loss results from the hair papilla being irreversibly damaged, deteriorated or dead. Hair receives its nutrients and life source from the small blood vessels that supply blood to the papilla (see pg. 75. Once the papilla degenerates, the follicle can no longer produce hair. Temporary hair loss is reversible and the hair is expected to grow back. Several things will cause intermediate and temporary hair loss, such as physical damage to the hair shaft, medication or systemic malfunctions.

Physically mistreating the hair shaft has no effect on the hair papilla. Hair that has been cut off, ruined, burned by excessive heat pressing, deteriorated from bleaching and other harsh chemicals will grow back if the process does not affect the scalp or hair papilla. Even if hair was to break off down to less than 1/8", the growth process initiated within the follicle (below the skin) is not impeded. This type of hair loss can be resolved by changing the behavior that is causing the hair to weaken and break off. Medication, drugs and chemicals can also cause intermediate hair loss. This may be a side effect that will go away once the substance is no longer administered in the body. Most drugs that interfere with blood circulation, hormones, and dividing cells will cause a change in the hair texture and its growth rate. Be mindful that each person's body is different and will have a different reaction to medication, drugs and treatments that have the known side effect of hair loss or thinning. The technical term for abnormal hair loss is Alopecia.

There are different types of alopecia:

Traction Alopecia is hair loss due to excessive pulling of the hair, such as tight braiding, rubber bands, hair rollers and barrett's.

Alopecia prematura is abnormal hair loss earlier than age 30.

Alopecia totalis is complete baldness.

Alopecia areata is bald spots in round patches. This condition is sudden and may be caused by damage to the nervous system, anemia, syphilis, and depressed blood circulation.

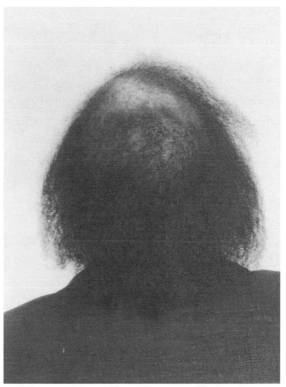

More and more females are suffering from permanent hair loss.

Problems with the reproductive system

The Gonad (sex glands) are a vital system of organs that regulate many body functions. When these glands are not functioning properly or removed, others areas of the body are affected, including the healthy growth of hair. Estrogen, a naturally produced hormone, is essential to the female well being. The absence of this hormone can cause the body to take on menopausal symptoms like hot flashes, heart palpitations, weight gain, skin problems and hair thinning. Hysterectomy (which should be avoided by all means) is the removal of the uterus and/or ovaries, which causes a loss of estrogen.[8] Some females have been lead to believe that female hair loss is normal and hereditary from fathers who have MPB (male pattern balding). Male pattern balding is directly proportional to age and is largely a function of the male hormone dihydotestosterone (DHT), the active form of testosterone. When the DHT comes in contact with the hair follicle it can stunt the growth and life cycle of the hair. This pattern of hair loss is hereditary for males but not females because we have different hormones.

Although the male hormone is the culprit for male pattern hair loss, the female hormone estrogen can affect the female order including hair growth. A disorder such as fibroids within the female reproductive system can interfere with the hair. Fibroids are muscle tumors that originate in the wall of the uterus and grow under the influence of estrogen. Estrogen regulates their growth, the more estrogen the faster they grow. It is believed that fibroids begin to grow because of an error in the gene that controls the rate of replication for uterine muscle cells. For reasons no one understands, fibroids are more commonly found in African-American and Jewish women.[9] Fibroids are believed to be inherited. If some females in your family have them, you may be predisposed to them. As it relates to hair, I have noticed in my clients who have fibroids, hysterectomy or other sex gland problems, there is a pattern of hair thinning. Usually the front top crown and the temple areas of the hair thin, feel dry or grow slower than normal. I have been able to encourage hair growth for my clients who sought my help at the early stages of thinning. My treatment program consists of reflexology massage, customized scalp care to stimulate hair growth in cases where the papilla is alive; diet and lifestyle change, and natural hair styling to preserve the hair that remains.

Chemotherapy and Some Medications

Clients often ask what exactly causes hair to come out during their chemo treatments and can it be prevented? Even though all patients do not lose their hair during chemotherapy treatments, there is no sure way to prevent it from happening at all. The human body is made up of millions of cells that have specific functions for life. There are two kinds of cells, single cells and dividing cells. The mass of layers of cells making hair tissue is made up of dividing cells. Since hair cells have a limited life span they must be replaced on a continuous basis. Cell division makes this happen. Cancer cells are mutations of dividing cells. This is how they reproduce at a rapid rate and spread throughout the body. When cancer is throughout the body it is impossible to locally destroy it. This is where chemotherapy comes in. Chemotherapy simply means "chemical therapy." During this therapy a chemical is administered to circulate through the body, hopefully to kill the dividing cancer cells. However, this chemical cannot distinguish between the good cells and the cancerous cells, making the good cells vulnerable to being destroyed in the treatment. This chemical only affects dividing cells. When the dividing hair cells are destroyed in the treatment, the hair does not reproduce. The result is that hair will fall out and not replace itself during the chemo treatment period. This is one of the side effects of this poisonous chemical. If you need to have chemotherapy, you can anticipate your hair falling out within three to four treatments. The dosage and particular drug will determine this. Consult your oncologist about your treatment and the side effect of hair loss.

As traumatic as this is for the chemo patient, the good news is that hair will usually grow back once the treatments are stopped. My clients who have lost all their hair during chemotherapy have grown back heads full of hair. In some cases the hair texture may come back thicker than before the treatment. Steroids also cause intermediate hair loss. Some medications prescribed for migraine headaches cause the hair to thin, change color and even bald.

Lupus

Lupus is a disease that generally affects women. It is a chronic inflammatory disease where the body's immune system attacks itself, unlike the AIDS virus that destroys the immune system. Clients with lupus often suffer hair loss. Usually the medication they are taking, such as steroids, shuts down the body's own adrenal hormone production. The toxic drugs used to treat this disease can also affect the dividing cells that produce hair. One client in particular had considerable hair growth once we regularly massaged the scalp and braided her hair. She is limited in braid style selections mostly because she has some areas that are very fine and cannot hold the weight of extension braids. At first we designed wigs for her hair loss, but the braid style and hair weave seem to encourage the most growth. Each client who has lupus will have a different hair loss pattern, scalp discoloration or disfiguration; therefore it is important to have a professional hair care stylist analyze the hair texture and strength to decide what style is safe and does not weaken the already fragile hair and sensitive scalp. Consult your doctor or other patients who may be able to give you ideas and recommendations for salons that treat hair loss conditions. However, keep in mind some doctors may be insensitive to female hair loss but don't let this discourage you. Talk to female nurses, patients and others for recommendations. I realize how important it is for you to look in the mirror and feel good about yourself, this is a part of the healing process; so don't give up; God will answer your prayers.

Naturally Thinning Hair

A short hair cut and tapered small styles are perfect for thinning hair conditions. If the hair is thin and lengthy it will appear thinner. For thinning fragile hair you do not need to add hair extensions. If your hair texture has changed due to medication, but has enough coverage to still wear it; have your stylist cut your hair into a "chic" short cut. Only you will know that it is thinner than your normal hair texture.

Another option to cover thin and bald areas of the head are selected braid styles. The objective is to create a style that camouflages the bald area but does not add any stress or tension to it. The stress and tension would come from starting a cornrow at the weak point of the hair loss area, or the weight of a hair extension braid that could break the already fragile hair. For a thin front hair line or bald sides, select a hair style where the braids cover the weak thin area. Never braid the hair back off the face; rather use a page boy style or curve braids on the weak hair line to protect it.

For a bald crown but strong edges, any style that does not part through the middle will cover this area of baldness. The ideal design should create the cornrows to braid through the bald spot. Even though the cornrow will not attach to the bald area, it will cover it.

If the nape area is thin or bald, braid a style that hangs to the back or is a low pin up style that covers the nape line. Styles such as a bun, straight back hanging or a low inverted braid can cover the bald nape area.

Styles for hair loss conditions

In the event of being permanently bald or having thinning hair, there are ways and styles that can help you live with the problem. Prevention is always the best option; however, for some, it is too late to consider due to medical circumstances. In the case of some medical therapy treatments, hair loss is inevitable so early preparation may make the process less frightening and depressing. It is helpful to prepare yourself psychologically for hair loss. This is where a natural hair stylist, experienced in wig styling and hair extensions, is most valued. I have even customized hair pieces to create hairlines for women who are bald from the front hairline to the top crown.

During cancer and other diseases, pain and nausea are felt but are invisible to another person. Only the person with the disease knows. However, hair loss is a visible reminder of the illness. It can be one of the most traumatizing and stressful side effects of treatment. A study was done that showed that often African-American women decide not to get recommended chemotherapy cancer treatments because of the one known side affect of losing their hair, despite knowing other treatments may not destroy the cancerous cells. Again, they risk their health because of fear of losing their hair. It has been proven that when patients look good they feel better, so to lose your hair is a double-blow from the illness. There are ways to cover temporary hair loss and make that part of the treatment less depressing. I recommend to clients, who know in advance they will experience hair loss, to buy a wig before they begin taking chemotherapy or other medications. This gives them comfort and time to focus on selecting a wig suitable to their face shape and style.

When choosing a wig, select one that looks natural; not too full, straight, stiff or shiny. Have your stylist cut it into a style to suit your face. Think of the wig as a new head of hair that needs to be cut and styled. You may buy a wig that gives you a totally new style or one that closely resembles your natural hair. One very young client (13 years old), had been coming to the salon to have her hair cornrowed. When she started her chemotherapy treatments I designed a wig in the exact cornrow style she had worn. She felt comfortable having a wig that was suitable for her age and the same style she had worn. A problem for children (African-American especially) who lose their hair during the chemotherapy treatments is difficulty in finding a wig that looks like a child's style and fits well. Having to wear a wig that is obvious and wiggy looking is an emotional downer to anyone's self-esteem and recovery.

Human hair wigs can be styled in a variety of looks. The advantage is that they are easy to curl and create the texture you may want. Although more costly and difficult to find, it is the best type wig if you like to curl and restyle your hair. A human hair wig can cost $55 dollars and up. Synthetic wigs are less costly and most abundant; however, it takes a good eye and good touch to find the best quality that looks like real hair. Fortunately, there is a large selection of synthetic wigs, and they, too, can be cut to suit your face shape. The better quality synthetic wigs can cost $25 dollars and up. Today, wigs are made with light weight caps so they do not have to be heavy and hot.

Look for wigs that are sewn in thin wefts, where space is between each row or hand tied, to allow the scalp to breath. There are also custom wigs for complete baldness.

Tips on selecting a natural looking and comfortable wig

1. Try to choose a wig that is close to your hair color and texture so that it does not give a drastic change.
2. If you still have some hair along the front hairline, leave it out so that your hair line gives the wig a very natural appearance.
3. If you are completely bald and the wigs feels like it may slide, attach a piece of adhesive wig tape to keep it stable, or have a custom wig made to fit.
4. Wigs can be cut to style or custom made for your hair and style needs.
5. Purchase two wigs; one for everyday wear and the other for special occasions.
6. Human hair wigs will generally last about six months with daily wear; synthetic wigs will last up to four months.
7. The wig should fit comfortably, feel lightweight and look fresh.
8. When the wig becomes matted, dull and dry looking it is time to shampoo (human hair) or discard (synthetic).
9. Braided wigs may feel heavier than loose hair wigs.
10. Avoid holding sprays and oil sheen sprays; these make the wig look shinny and artificial.

Hair weaves are not recommended for total baldness or if the hair is extremely fine and fragile. Because the foundation of the weave is a cornrow, the client's hair must be strong enough to braid and anchor wefts of hair onto. The hair weave is best suited for chemically damaged hair or small areas of permanent bald spots. The bald spots must have strong hair around the spots perimeter in order to secure the hair extension over it. Many clients who have bald crowns from medications (high blood pressure, diabetes, scar tissue from chemical burns) choose the weave because it is not hot, easy to sleep in, can be worn while exercising, and combs and styles like your own hair.

Hats and Head Wraps

I believe in having several wonderful hats in your wardrobe. This is another way to cover hair loss or a bad hair day. If the weather is very hot, a straw hat or cotton wrap may be cool and more comfortable than a wig. And of course the cold winter chill can be avoided with a nice, natural fiber, winter hat.

Scarves and head wraps are also a great alternative to cover the head. They are fashionable and quite comfortable. If this is new to you, buy a large piece of cotton fabric and practice wrapping and tying the head wrap. The key to wrapping the hair is to criss-cross the scarf ends and loosely tuck the fabric to secure a shape. Position the wrap away from the face.

Today, there is no reason for a woman to have to walk around with baldness. There are many safe and natural looking style options that comfortably cover this hair problem. The biggest challenge is finding a stylist who specializes in this method of hair care and can promise that their styles for hair loss will not further encourage hair damage to the existing or growing hair.

BODY SIGNS ——— What to look for.

The body has its way of giving us visible signs when we lack the necessary foods and elements for good health. I can look at a clients eyes, teeth, hair and fingernails to determine overall health and wellness.

Eyes are the window to the brain so they should be clear and white. If they are dirty looking, blood shot and spotty, the person may be lacking vitamin A, potassium, or have a toxic liver. Drink plenty of carrot juice and fast to cleanse the body. Include more raw fruits and vegetables into the diet.

Teeth and gum decay are warning signs that the body is toxic. This condition will also poison other organs and healthy parts of the body via the blood stream. Rotten teeth and pyorrhea of the gums are the most obvious signs of oral hygienic neglect. Place papaya tablets in each side of the mouth to break down the dead gum tissue for pyorrhea.[10] Do this daily until you see improvement. Practice good oral hygiene and make regular visits to the dentist and periodontist.

Finger nails are a window to see your blood circulation. Moons on each nail indicate good circulation. No moons means poor circulation and a lot of mucus in the body.

Skin is one of the eliminatory organs. Bad skin is an indication that the body is toxic, too acidic, has poor digestion, is diseased or in urgent need for internal cleansing and nutritional building. All the creams, acne prescriptions and outside cosmetic care will not help the internal problems of the body.

Hair is the one part of the body that women will quickly seek help for styling. It belongs to our body and is a clue that the body is in optimum wellness or malfunctioning and deficient. It is external evidence that can lead to the solution of a problem. Balding, thinning, brittle hair, certain graying, and scalp disorders are some of the indications that the body is breaking down. Getting to know your hair and its relationship to your body combined with other health care regimens will help the hair tremendously, promising you a full healthy head of hair for life.

Nutrition and Nourishment

As a natural hair care stylist I can offer a book full of styles and beauty ideas for healthy hair; however, there is nothing more essential to good hair than good food. What you eat, what you put into your body that nourishes it or may rob it of nourishment is key to your overall hair growth. Something as basic as a healthy diet may make the difference in the health and beauty of your hair, skin and nails. Sometimes women may ask other women where they go to get their hair styled, because it looks so healthy; when the real question should be "what is your diet?" The beauty of another woman's hair can simply depend on how and what she eats. She may live off a diet rich in organic fresh fruits, vegetables, grains, seeds, sprouts, and water, while your daily intake may consist of coffee and donuts, cheeseburgers, colas, fried chicken, potato chips, alcohol and cigarettes.

Live foods are imperative to your wellness and pretty hair. Lack of vitamins and life giving elements will cause deterioration, disease, and illness. Some women may live a life of mal-nourishment and keep a head full of hair, but the deterioration may show up in another form of dis-ease. If your hair is in poor health and bad condition, this may very well be a warning to improve your diet.

A well balanced daily diet should consist of:

- *Fresh fruits and vegetables* Select in season, tree-ripe local produce. Fruits are body cleaners. Best eaten in the morning and throughout the day. Vegetables are body builders that provide the necessary vitamins for strength.
- *Carbohydrates* Some complex carbohydrates are vegetables, whole grains, beans, pasta, oats, corn, dates, figs, potatoes, and bran. They provide the body with warmth and energy. Fiber foods. Avoid too much consumption of simple carbohydrates, i.e. sugars, candy, pastry etc..
- *Proteins* Protein is found in dried beans, lentils, grains, millets, nuts, animal protein, eggs, fish, dairy products, soy, apricots, avocados, figs, olives, and fresh beans. Proteins are needed for building and repairing the body (For complete protein, eat a meal of brown rice and beans)
- *Minerals* They are needed for the formation of healthy bones and teeth, controlling the body fluids and keeping the nervous system healthy. Minerals trigger the enzyme process in the body. Your body needs up to twenty-nine trace minerals, such as zinc, copper, mercury, lead; and 12 major minerals.

The 12 major minerals are — Calcium, Chlorine, Fluorine, Iodine, Iron, Magnesium , Manganese, Phosphorus, Potassium, Silicon, Sodium, Sulphur

• Calcium is essential for the formation of strong bones and teeth, prevents bone loss and helps many other vital body functions. It enables the body to repair, rebuild and heal. The following foods are high in calcium: molasses, green leafy vegetables, broccoli, cabbage, buttermilk, dried figs, fish, milk, okra, cottage cheese, natural grain cereals, seeds, nuts.

• Chlorine is the element for cleansing the body. It keeps the juices flowing in the body. Chlorine foods include spinach, cabbage, celery, figs, tomatoes, dates, beans, carrots, milk, fish.

• Fluorine is a much needed element to resist dis-ease like colds, flu, and bronchial infections. This element is found in raw foods that include green leafy tops of vegetables, nuts, goat milk, and green quince. Cooking destroys fluorine in foods.

• Sulphur provides the body with heat, protects the protoplasm of cells, and disinfects the blood. Winter vegetables are a source of sulphur; these vegetables have their own source of heat to grow in the cold. You can get sulphur from brussel sprouts, kale, cauliflower, broccoli, onions, turnips and cabbage.

• Iodine foods are needed for a healthy thyroid. Iodine foods include sea vegetables, kelp, dulse, arame, kombu, fish, garlic, mushrooms, chard, beans, sea salt.

• Iron is the element for good blood and oxygen. It is needed for energy and circulation to draw oxygen from the air into the body and to keep you from becoming anemic. Without it we cannot exist. You can find iron in natural black strap molasses, greens, fish, liver, lima beans, kidney beans, soybeans, pumpkins, raisins, prunes, peaches, almonds, dates, beets, rice, pears. *Brittle thin hair and baldness are signs of iron deficiency.*

• Magnesium is the body calming element that is needed for healthy nervous and muscle systems. It is stored in the bowels and indispensable to enzyme activity. This element is found in many foods including yellow vegetables, cornmeal, seaweed, green leafy vegetables, seafood, apples, black-eyed peas, lima beans, garlic, brown rice, brewer's yeast and bananas.

• Manganese is the element that keeps you in balance and with "love." It is a brain and nerve element, aids in the formation of mother's milk, regulates blood sugar, and is essential to healthy nervous and immune systems. Nuts and seeds are high in manganese. Black walnuts, avocados, seaweed, vegetables, pineapples, salads, blueberries, legume's and whole grains are great sources.

• Phosphorus is found in most foods including fish, eggs, asparagus, corn, dairy products, garlic, nuts, seaweed, and whole grains. This element is necessary for cell growth, bone formation, brain nourishment and the conversion of food to energy.

• Potassium is a great healer and body alkalizer. It helps to regulate heart rhythm, water balance in the body, and muscle contraction and carries nutrients to the cells. Bee pollen, potato skin broth, bananas, figs, winter squash, yams, avocados, and garlic are high in potassium.

• Silicon is the binding magnetic element that carries messages from the brain to different organs in the body. We need this element for formation of connective tissue, a vital nervous system, healthy skin and hair. Hair is a reserve where silicon is stored. With a good silicon reserve, you will feel improvement in the hair. The best sources for silicon are skins and peelings of vegetables, oat straw, alfalfa, sprouts, bell peppers, leafy green vegetables, cucumber juice and whole grains.

• Sodium can be found in most foods. The best sodium is biochemical from plant life. Whey contains a high level of natural sodium. It is needed to keep the joints limber and young, and the proper water balance and blood pH level of 7.5. Sodium should be balanced with potassium.

Pure, natural, live plants, grains and (for some) flesh are essential for a wholesome diet to wellness. Whether or not you eat flesh, your daily diet should include 60% fresh raw fruits and vegetables, whole grains, carbohydrates, clean water and fresh air.

Hair Food Recipes

These foods are loaded with hair nourishing vitamins and minerals.

Black strap molasses drink (cold)
Mix:1 teaspoon organic molasses into
8 ounces of mineral water or sparkling water
1 teaspoon of maple syrup (optional)

Hot molasses drink (Replace your cup of coffee)
1 teaspoon of molasses
Cup of hot distilled water

Brewers yeast drink
Mix 1 teaspoon brewers yeast into
8oz. of fresh squeezed orange juice, carrot juice or yogurt drink

Alfalfa sprouts salad
Bowl of sprouts
1 large vine ripe tomato (diced up)
Season with olive oil, garlic powder and kelp

Sea vegetables, sea weeds (high in protein and contains all trace minerals)
Use for seasoning, put on sandwich, mix in soups, gravies, salads
sushi wrap or eat as a side vegetable. (Nori, Kombu, Dulse, Arame, Kelp)

Vitamin B_6 Salad
Watercress
Pecans
Seaweeds
Grille tuna slices
A hint of dill yogurt dressing (mix fresh dill into plain yogurt, season with Spike)

Iced Horsetail tea (great source of silicon for the hair)
Horsetail tea (equivalent to 6 tea bags) 1 teabag of green tea
Quart of distilled water
Tablespoon of fresh squeezed ginger
1/4 cup or more of Honey

Notes

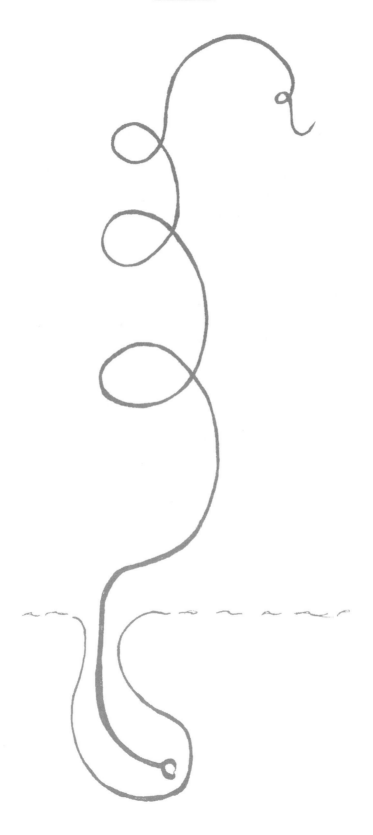

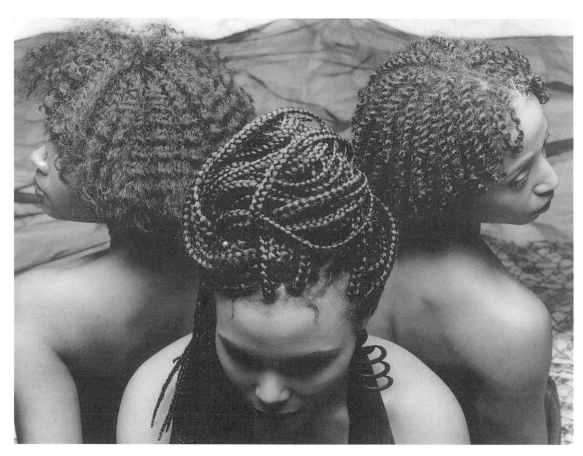

Braids, Twist and Weave

Natural Hair Care, Twists Locks Braids, and Weaves

5

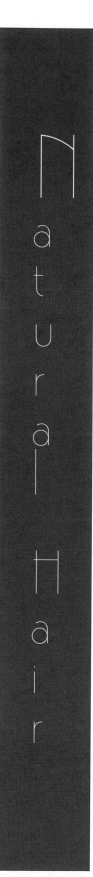

Natural Hair

Natural hair care and self-styling
Pamela Ferrell's easy shampoo, comb out and blow dry
The natural, styling with twist / twist-out texturing
How to find a natural hair care stylist

Natural hair care and self-styling

Most women who are at the mercy of their hair stylist become frustrated with their hair because they do not know how to do it themselves. Straightening the hair became popular not only for the sleek European look, but often because it made the black woman's hair seemingly easy to comb and manage. Yet, many women who straighten their hair still do not know what to do with it. They pull their easy-to-comb hair into one of the most popular do-it-yourself hair styles -- the ponytail.

An easy-to-comb ponytail can be created without using chemicals and natural hair offers so many other choices. Whether the hair is straight or curly is not the issue; the key is being able to comfortably work with your hair, learn new styles that suit its texture and keep it healthy.

I recommend that every woman learn self styling. It is a way to become familiar with your hair type and free yourself from depending on someone to always do your hair; someone who may not have your hair's best interest at heart. Knowing how to do your own hair gives you a voice in your hair care and where and when you will have someone else do it. Going to the beauty salon to care for your hair should be a choice, not a dependency.

Women who are not good at styling their own hair should know at least the basics; like shampooing, combing and one quick simple style. What if you should move to a new city or you're away from home and your hair needs care? God forbid, your hair stylist should move away, disappear or retire. What would happen if you lost your job and can no longer afford to go to the hair salon? For these and other reasons, it is imperative that you learn how to shampoo and care for your hair.

Every woman should be able to do at least one hair style herself. Self-styling is effortless if you learn the basics and just give it a try. "Do-it-yourself" hair styles can be a saving grace between salon visits or when you cannot get to the hair salon. Just keep three things in mind. First, remember that your hair's length and texture will determine how your style will look. Second, don't expect to do your favorite style perfectly on the first try. It will require practice and experimenting regularly. Third, don't give up so soon. It takes hair stylists years to become expert in styling hair. It will take you several weeks or months to become your own expert stylist.

I always suggest practicing self styling in the evening (in front of a mirror), when you have time and you're not trying to create the style for an outing. This will allow you to re-do the style as often as needed. For the styles that need to air dry, you can sit under a hood dryer for quick results. Also it is best to try these styles over the weekend until you have mastered them in a reasonable time.

To be sure the style is neat all over, use the mirror to check all views. Develop a good habit of looking at all angles of yourself when you are styling your own hair. Look at profiles, front, back and top crown. I have seen hair styles that are beautiful in the front but barely touched in the back. A hand mirror held up to a large stationary mirror will show all sides of the hair style.

Let's begin.

Always view all sides of a hair style:

1. To view the back of your head, stand with your back to a stationary mirror. To see the left side, stand with your left profile facing the mirror. For the right side, stand with your right profile facing the mirror and to see the top crown stand with your back to the stationary mirror, tilt your head back so that the crown faces the mirror.

2. Hold the hand mirror in front of you slightly to the left or right side, and look at the back, left, right and top crown of the head. Look into the small hand mirror to see the reflection in the stationary mirror.

Next, learn how to handle your hair and select the right tools for grooming and styling. The best tool that you will ever have for styling and handling the hair is your hands and fingers. You can separate the hair, smooth it, finger comb and shape it into interesting textures using your hands. Many of the natural styles do not need constant combing for styling and maintenance. The combs, brushes and hair dryers are mostly used for prepping and preparing the hair.

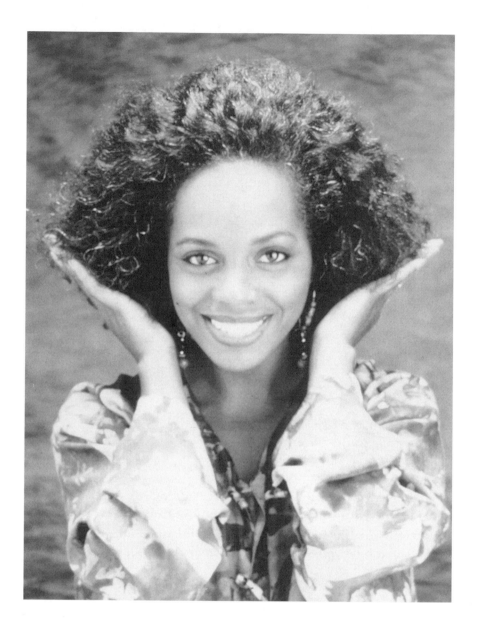

Are you using the right combs and styling tools? Try combing thick curly hair with a fine tooth comb, and you are likely to have a headache. The tools that you use for styling and grooming your hair will make a world of difference in how comfortable it feels. Often times women will cause breakage to the hair by pulling and yanking, trying to comb their curly hair with the wrong comb. It would be like combing straight hair with an afro pic, it just wouldn't work. For thick, curly hair, use a wide round-tooth comb. Plastic is the least costly and easy to find; however, for the naturalist, there are wood combs. Wood combs are very lightweight, will not cause static in the hair, but may not feel weighty enough to comb very thick hair. To complete your hair care vanity, certain tools are essential for grooming natural hair.

Hair pins and bobby pins What is the difference?
The bobby pin holds the hair flat and the hair pin is used to hold the hair full.

The *hair pin* has open ends. It is used to anchor a roll, bun, curl or loose hair in a stationary style. To anchor the hair properly without the hair pin irritating and touching the scalp slide the pin in half way and turn it in the opposite direction. To pin a roll, place the pin away from the roll hooking a part of it, then turn the pin into the roll hidden underneath but not touching the scalp. If your scalp itches or feels irritated by the plastic on the pin, replace the hair pin daily.

The *bobby pin*, has two prong ends that are closed. To pin the hair flat, hold the hair in place, open the bobby pin and slide it onto the hair.

Hair pin   *Bobby pin*

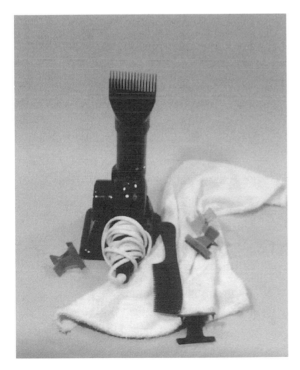

The basic styling tools for the shampoo, comb-out and blow dry process for natural hair

Large tooth comb - (Afro or volume) used to comb out thick curly hair.
All purpose comb - great for parting the hair and combing the hairline smooth.
Blow dryer with a pic comb nozzle - use to dry, loosen and smooth the hair.
Butterfly hair clamps - use to keep the hair separate while combing out.

Pamela Ferrell's easy shampoo, comb out, and blow dry for natural hair

Gather large towels, natural shampoo, hair conditioner, large-tooth comb, clamps, blow-dryer with a pic comb attachment.

Shampoo

1. Rinse the hair thoroughly, then apply lathered shampoo to the scalp and hair.

2. Massage the scalp with your fingers, using in and out motions. In a pulling motion, stretch the hair out to work the lather to the ends. Never scrub in circular motions.

3. Rinse, give a second shampoo, then rinse again thoroughly.

4. Towel squeeze the excess water from the hair, then apply a hair conditioner; leave the conditioner on up to 5 minutes, then rinse it out thoroughly.

5. Wrap the hair with a towel, then towel blot the hair to remove excess water.

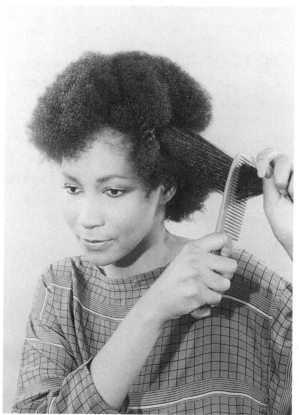

1.

Comb-out

(see photos 1-4)

1. Part the hair into sections about the size of your palm. Thick hair make 10-12 sections; fine thin hair make 4-6 sections.

2. With one hand, hold the hair close to the scalp, to prevent the hair from pulling while combing out the ends.

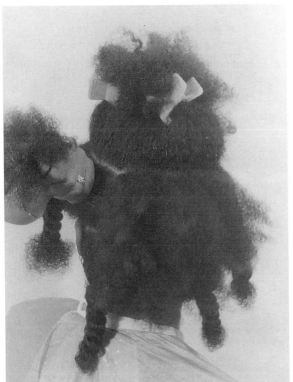

2.

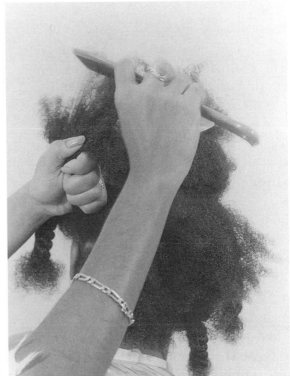

3.

3. Comb out the ends first, gradually combing down to the hair closest to the scalp. Comb in gentle plucking movements and never try to pull through a snarl because this will tighten the tangle. Stretch the hair ends outward as you comb.

4. Divide the combed out section into two pieces and loosely twist the hair. This organizes and separates the hair to make the blow-dry process easy. You can let the twisted hair air dry naturally for a textured effect or blow dry the hair after 15 to 30 minutes.

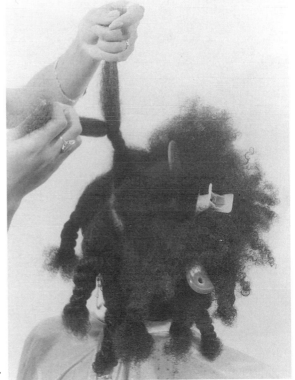

4.

Blow-dry

The blow-dry process is similar to the comb-out procedure. Use the comb nozzle attachment on the blow dryer to comb through and dry the hair.

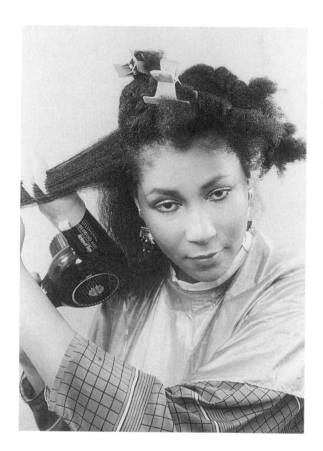

1. Starting at the nape area, untwist one section at a time, (for thick coarse, hair hold the hair close to the scalp; for softer texture hair stretch the hair outward) and blow dry the ends first.

2. While stretching the hair ends outward and <u>angling the air flow away from the scalp</u>, gradually work downward to the hair closest to the scalp. This will prevent the hot air from burning the scalp.

3. After blow drying each section, the natural hair should be smooth and easy to comb through.

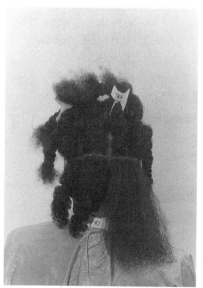
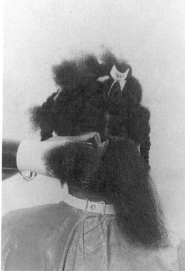
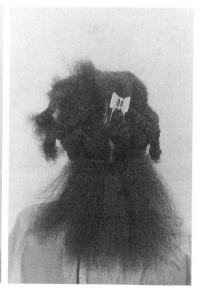

Smooth frizzy and puffy hairline edges

For natural styling, one important finishing touch is to smooth the hairline edges. This will give the style definition. All hair textures can be smooth around the hairline. Smoothing does not mean to straighten; it simply means to flatten the curl, kink, frizz or wispy hairs that frame the face. Some women may choose not to do this; however, the most frequent complaint I hear from black women about their hair is the frizzy, curly hairline that distracts from the rest of the hair style. This is one reason women feel the need to straighten their hair and think someone who has smooth edges has "good hair." All healthy hairlines, whether curly, kinky, wavy or straight, are considered good.

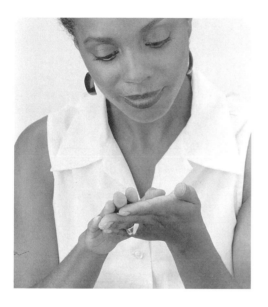

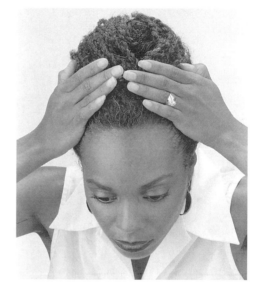

FRIZZIES

1. Rub the hands together with a dab of hair cream, or light gel.

2. Rub the moistened hands over the hairline directing frizzed hair back.

3. Firmly tie the moistened hairline with a cotton scarf. Leave on for 15 minutes or overnight. Once you remove the scarf the hairline is flat and smooth.

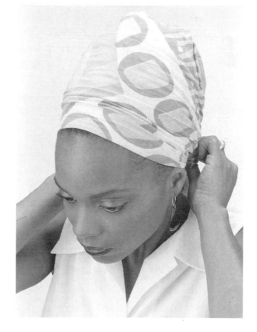

Classic Tuck with Curly Bang

Using a hair accessory helps to create perfect rolls and simple elegant up-styles. My Hair Tucker™ accessory eliminates the need to use hair pins. (Some women are sensitive to hair pins.) First, prepare the hair by blow drying or twist texturing to make it pliable and easy to tuck. Depending on your hair length, here are some do-it-yourself styles that can be created with a simple tuck.

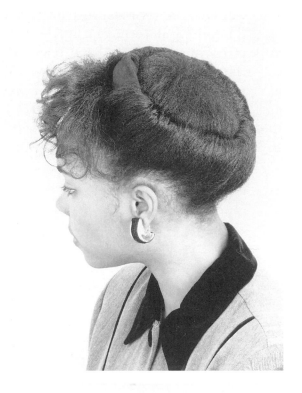

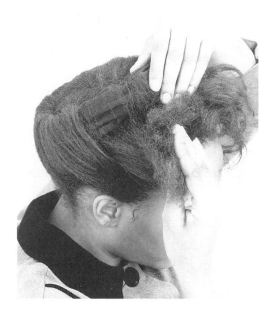

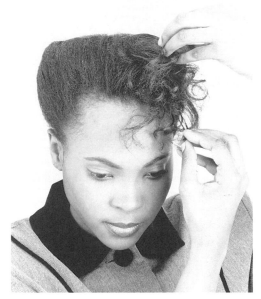

1. Comb the hair downward all around the face, place the Hair Tucker™ down over the crown with the hair hanging below.
2. Tuck the hair ends around the band to create a smooth roll. Leave out a small front section and curl the bang to softly frame the face.

Side Tuck

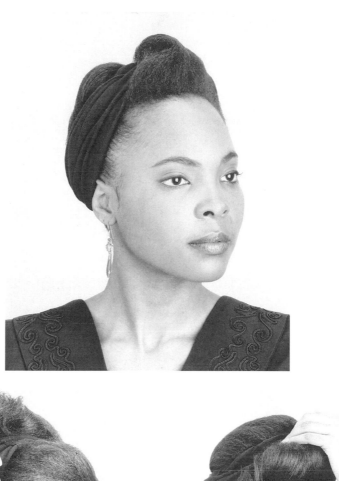

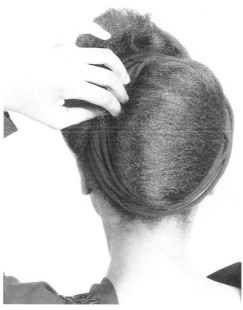

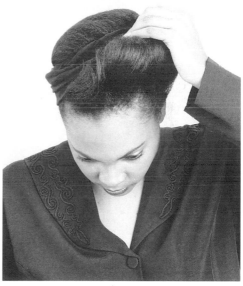

1. Comb the hair upward to one side. Place the Hair Tucker™ band over the back to one side hairline, on a diagonal from temple to opposite side behind the ear.
2. Tuck the side front section over the Hair Tucker™ band to cover and secure it. Shape the front hair with height and a soft wave.

Upstyle Tuck

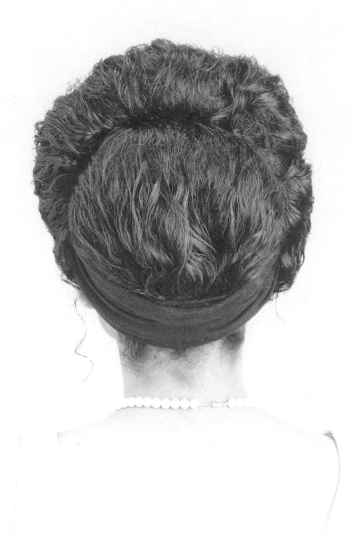

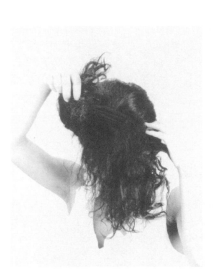

1. Comb the hair forward from the nape to the face.
2. Place the Hair Tucker™ band over the hair combed forward, leaving the front hair hanging free.
3. Tuck the front hair over the band toward the back to secure the Hair Tucker™ and create the height in the front.
4. To add softness to this elegant upstyle pull out strands of wispy hair along the hairline.

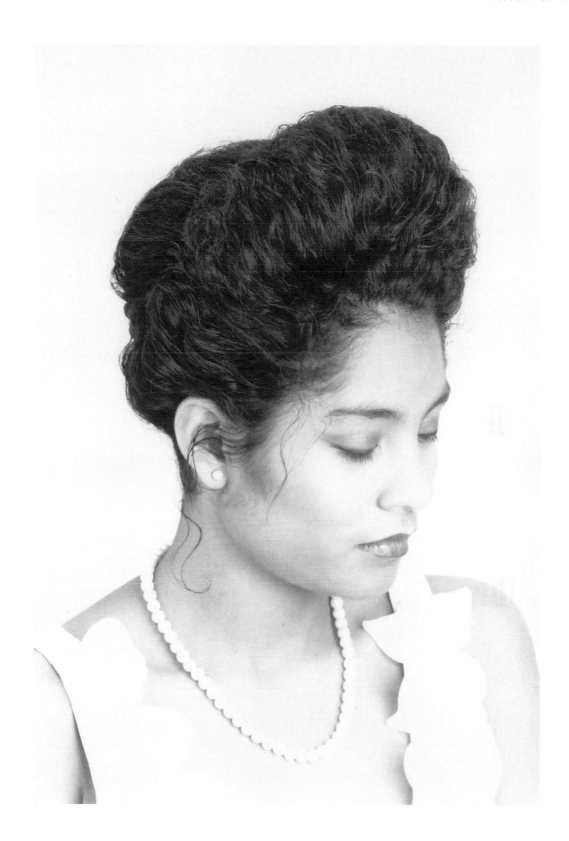

The Natural—Freedom Hair

Short, long, sculpted, full, round, flat top, mixed texture, and soft like cotton; the natural is here forever. There are so many ways to wear a natural. The various looks are determined by your hair length, texture, and how you groom it. You can wear your hair combed out to look like cotton, towel ruffled to create "pepper corn" curls or even glossy coils using the hand roll method. It all depends on how you work your natural hair. Now that you have learned about hair texture, choosing the right products and curl patterns, these things are important for keeping your natural soft, supple and gleaming. A complaint I often hear is that natural hair feels dry and looks dull. As you discover how to work with your hair you will realize that your true natural hair is soft and has a unique style of its own. Here are some tips on how to groom and maintain your natural.

For the *short natural*, shampoo and condition the hair as often as needed. Always moisten the hair with a mist of water before combing, to soften it. Use a large-tooth comb or pick. While the hair is moist, hand shape any straggly hairs in place. To keep the hair perfectly neat, regular trims are important. Depending on how fast your hair grows and how close the style is cut, a trim every three to six weeks is normal. If you are overdue for a trim or want to grow your natural longer, you can still keep it perfectly sculpted by hand shaping or molding it with a scarf. To mold the short natural with a scarf, moisten the hair, massage in an oil or creme for sheen, comb or pick it out, hand pat it in shape, then gently tie it flat with a large scarf. Leave the scarf on for 15 minutes, remove, and the natural will look neat and perfectly cut. To enhance your natural curl, wet your hair and massage in a natural gel pomade, rub the hair in circular motions to form curls, let air dry and do not comb.

For the *long full natural,* the key is to soften and loosen the hair so that it has body and does not feel brittle. To loosen the natural curl and modify your hair texture, shampoo, condition and lightly oil the hair, do a texture set such as a twist knot wet set, flat twist, individual twist or soft braids. Allow the hair to dry thoroughly. Finger comb the hair into shape. For a soft, fluffy, cottony "fro," comb the hair out thoroughly, shake it and let it fall into place. Keep the ends trimmed or clipped as needed. To add a special touch to your natural, individual twist or hand roll the perimeter. The difference between today's natural and the sixties Afro is the creativity of mix-media styling and shaping.

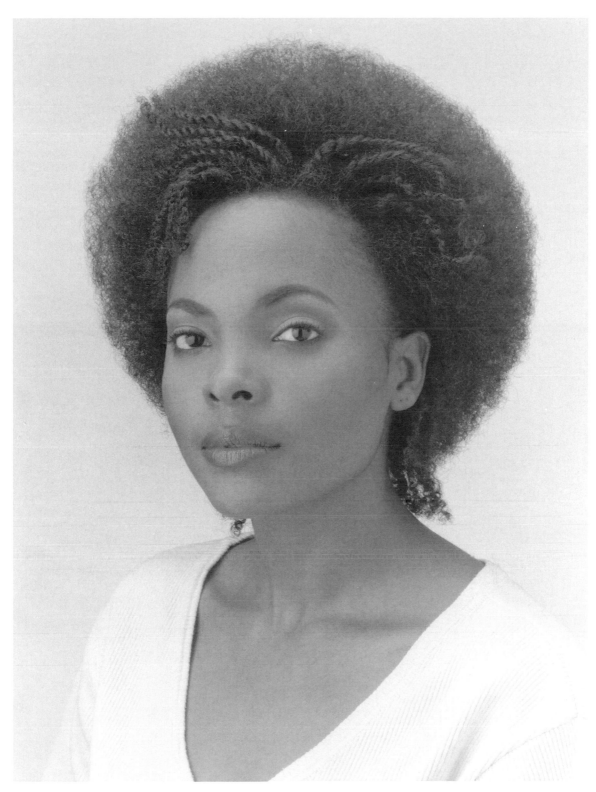

Mix-media natural

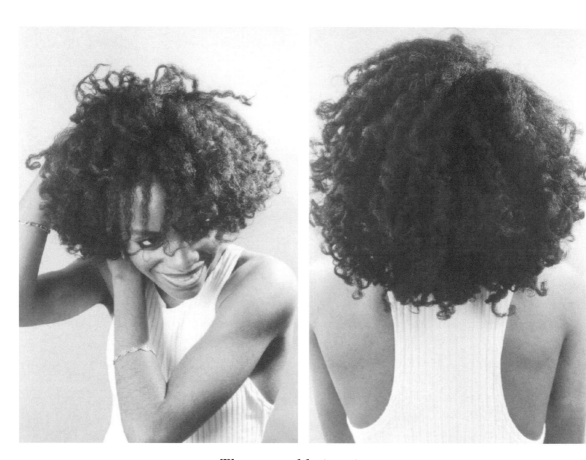

The natural hair twistout.

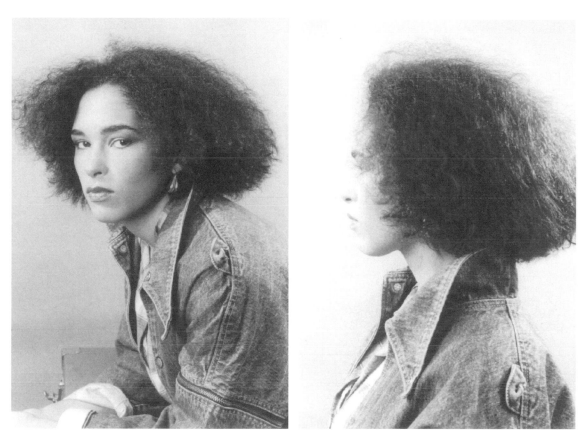

The natural hair softly blow dried.

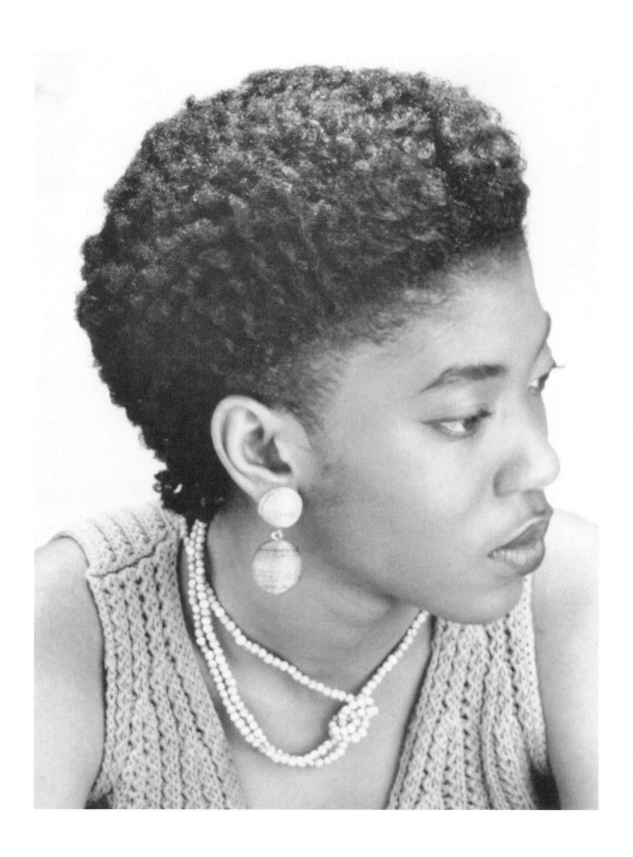

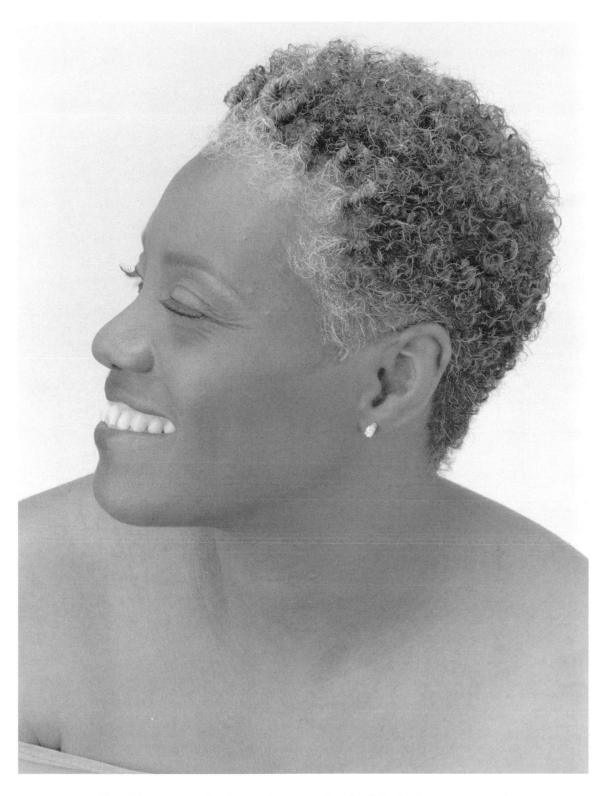

To add texture and enhance the natural curl, while the hair is wet, apply
a light gel and handroll the front hairline.

Twist knot wet set

1. After a shampoo, thoroughly comb out the hair and part it in sections about the size of your palm.

2. Divide the section in two and loosely twist the hair to the very end, then fold and tuck the end inside the base of the twist section. Make up to 12 sections.

3. Tie a scarf around the hair-line to smooth the edges and let the twisted hair air dry.

4. Once the hair has dried, loosen the twists and using the fingers, separate the twists and arrange the hair in the desired shape and style. To add more texture to the hair line, add twists at the front hairline or add twists throughout the interi-or of the style.

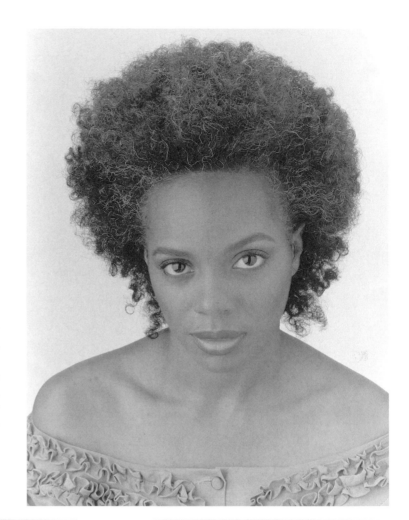

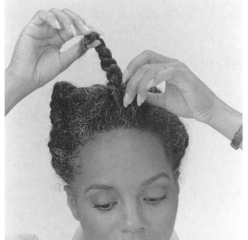

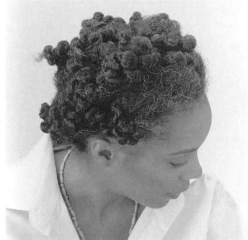

"Crown Puff"

This quick and easy pull up or pull back style is a classic. It can be done after the hair has been textured with the twist knot wet set. You can use a decorative fabric band, a Hair Tucker™ or a comb barrette to pull the hair away from the face into a soft afro puff on the crown or at the back of the head. For style variations, shape the hair even or finger pic it for an uneven texture. (pg. 125)

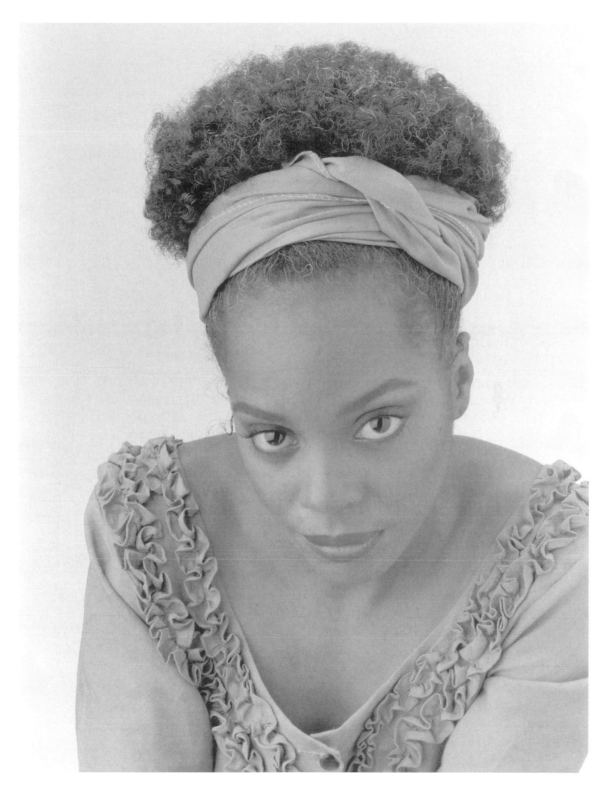

Natural hair textured with the twist knot wet set.

Styling with Twist

The twist style is going to replace pressing combs and chemical straightening for black women's hair. For the woman who wears natural hair, it is the long sought-after solution to maintaining curly, kinky hair. If you learn to use this style, you will never again feel the need to straighten your hair. It helps to minimize the bulk of thick hair, re-defines the hairs natural curl, and makes the hair manageable from day to day.

The initial twisting takes time, but be patient with yourself; the more you do this style the faster you will get. Eventually, you can do it without a mirror, while relaxing to your favorite music or movie. This will make the time go by quickly. Even though one to two hours seems like a long time, it is time well spent for a hair style that can last up to two weeks or longer with a shampoo and once it is done, styling the hair is quick, easy and predictable.

It will cut down the 30 to 60 minutes you may spend each day fooling with your hair. Grooming and styling natural twisted hair gives you more options and style variety. The size of the twist, wet styling or heat styling all change the appearance and flexibility of the style. Very small twists can be easily curled and styled in many different ways like loose hair. The larger twist will give the hair a lock-style appearance. Once the hair is twisted, it can be worn hanging or softly gathered and pinned in place.

The individual twist style is the most gentle style for kinky, curly hair types. With it you can wear contemporary styles, wet & curly, or stationary styles, where every hair strand stays in place. However, unlike the extension styles, it does require regular re-styling or bi-weekly visits to the salon.

The twist is similar to a braid except two pieces of hair are used instead of three. The distinct difference between them is that it takes less time to do twist styles, and the twist feels soft and looks fuller. There are two methods of twisting the hair -- the flat twist, which is like a cornrow, and the individual twist, which is like a plait. The flat twist lays along the scalp and is stationary; the individual twist extends from the scalp and can be rotated in a circle, giving the hair the most versatility and style flexibility. And of course the two methods can be combined to give a style movability or permanent position where needed. Even though there are twist styles that can be done using hair extensions, they do not curl like natural hair, nor do they resemble the unique beauty of the natural twist and are difficult to do yourself.

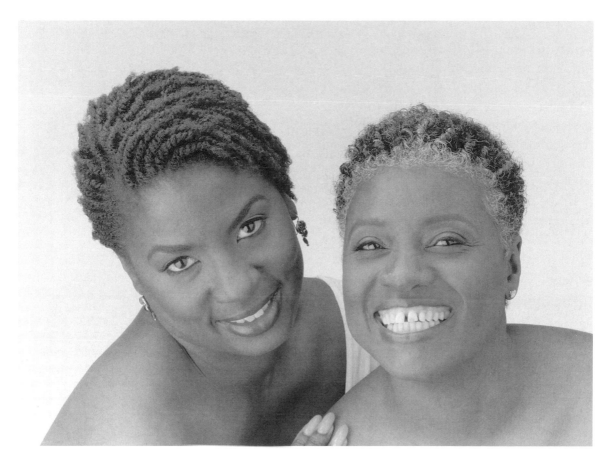

For a total new look, shampoo and wet style the individual twists. Usually after the shampoo, the hair will coil and shrink, making the style shorter. For certain styles, like the twist out with curly ends, the shrinkage is preferred. Women who like to shampoo and comb their hair frequently choose the twist style over extension braids and corn-rows. It gives the natural hair freedom.

If you decide to twist your own hair, time and patience are needed. The amount of time it takes to do your entire head in individual twists will depend on your hair length, texture and the size of the curl. On an average, it may take a professional hair braider up to two hours to do regular size individual twists. If you are planning to twist your own hair, initially it may take you longer than the professional braider. Plan to take an extra 30 minutes or longer until you improve your time. Depending on the effect you want, you may twist your hair while it is wet, air dried or blown straight. Each process will give a very different effect.

How to individually twist your hair

1. Starting at the nape area, part a small rounded section of hair.
2. Divide the section into two even parts and criss-cross the hair gently to create the twist. Twist size is determined by the section size and amount of tension (tight or loose) used to twist the hair.
3. To secure the ends, twist the hair small to the end. The hair ends must be kinky/curly and not straight or cut even. 4. To set the natural curl in the hair, wet the hands with water and moisten the ends of the twist or use a spray bottle and mist the ends with water.
5. Other finishing options are to set the hair on sponge rollers for 30 minutes, hot curl, steam set or just let them hang straight.

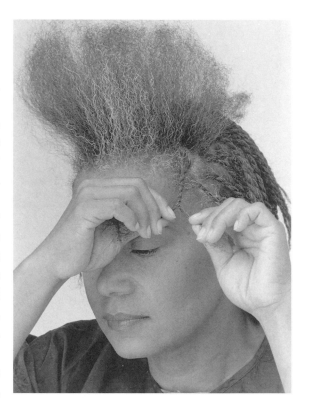

Wet Twist
When you twist the hair wet it gives a coily curly effect.

1. After a shampoo and conditioning, apply a light oil, and pre-section long hair into 4-6 sections; hair 4" or shorter can be twisted without pre-sectioning. Starting at the nape area, part a small rounded section of hair.

2. Apply a small amount of pomade gel and divide the section into two even parts and criss-cross the hair gently to create the twist. The hair will coil and curl as you twist.

Note: *If you twist wet hair, the hair may air dry during the process making the wet and dry twists look slightly different. To prevent this, re-moisten the hair as you work.*

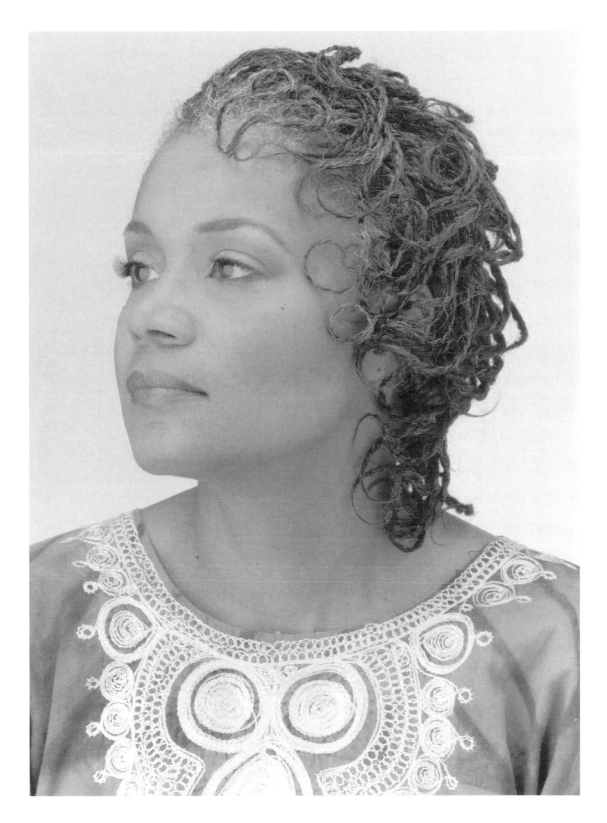

Dry twisting

If you individually twist hair after it has air dried in the twist knot wet set (pg. 124), it will give a full curly style as if the hair was rolled.

1. After shampooing and conditioning the hair, apply a light oil, comb out and part the hair in 8-10 sections. Divide each section in two, twist loosely and tuck the end of the twist inside the base of the section.
2. After the hair completely air dries, untwist each large section and individually twist the hair in small twists. The hair will curl as you twist it.

Blow dry and twist

For long, sleek, straight twist, blow dry the hair smooth.

Blow drying the hair makes it effortless to comb thick hair and easy to make uniform sections for straight twist. Also, the blow dry process can be a relief for hair that has been handled frequently in its wrinkled state. If the hair is easy to comb and section during twisting, it will not break as you handle it. (Note: the straight twist will coil up once the hair is wet again)

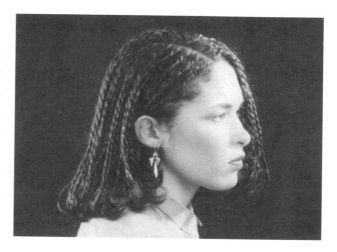

1. Shampoo and blow dry the hair smooth.
2. Starting at the nape and working up to the front, twist small evenly parted sections.
3. Twist small at the ends and leave to hang straight or curl the ends.

Three week twist style

The individual twist style can be worn up to three weeks and styled differently each week. At bedtime, wear a Hair Tucker™ or scarf to preserve the style and hold the shape. In the morning, shake the hair and moisten, if needed, to re-shape the style. Even though the individual twist style can last longer than three weeks, it is discouraged because the hair will tangle and begin to lock.

1. *Week one* -- Blow dry and individual twist the hair. Curl the ends for a hanging style. To maintain the curl, use hot rollers instead of curling irons. (Direct heat from hot irons can scorch the hair ends.)

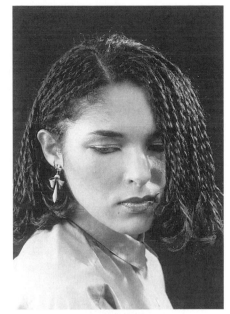

2. *Week two* -- Shampoo or just wet the hair lightly to spiral curl the ends. Wear hanging the first few days. Once you wet the twist you must moisten the hair every morning to freshen the curl and reshape the twist style to hang neatly in place. Apply oil for a sheen and tie the edges to smooth the hair. If you get tired of wearing the hair hanging, pin up the twists. You may also roll the twists on large sponge rollers to give body while keeping the coily texture.

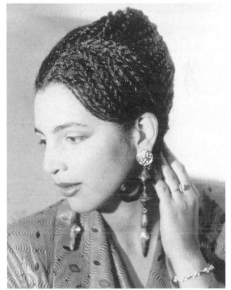

3. *Week three* -- Shampoo the hair with the individual twists in, apply a light gel or oil for sheen to smooth the edges. After the hair has completely air dried, wear in a pin-up style or untwist and wear the twist out. The twist out will add longevity to the individual twist style and give volume and a totally new look.

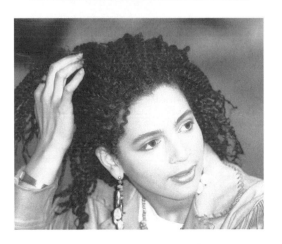

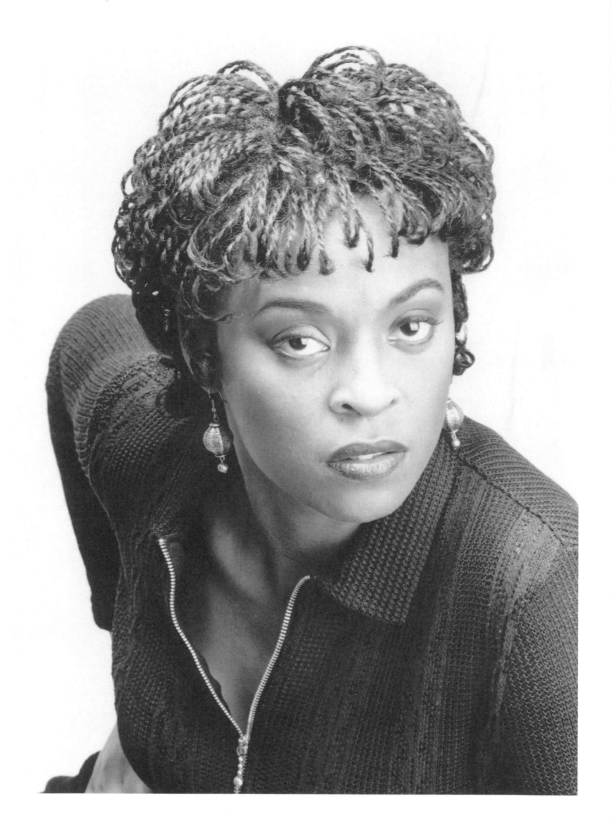

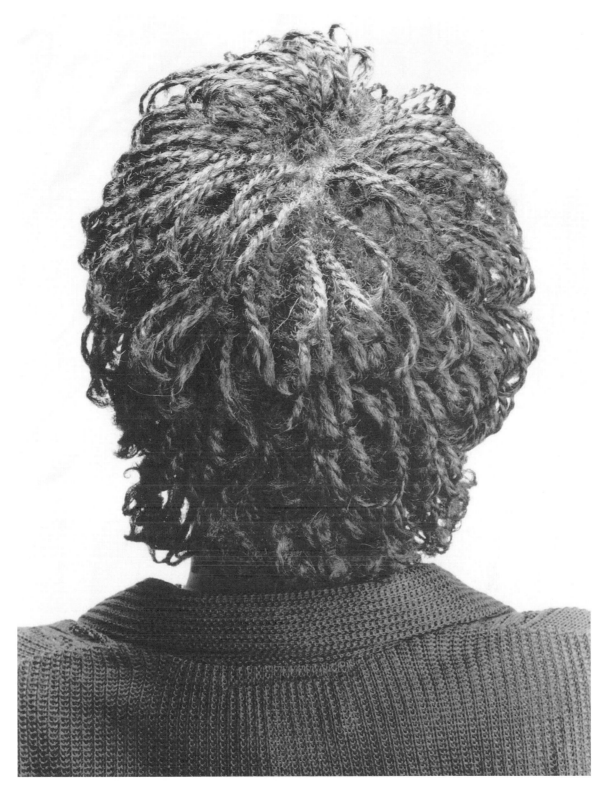

Individual twist curled.

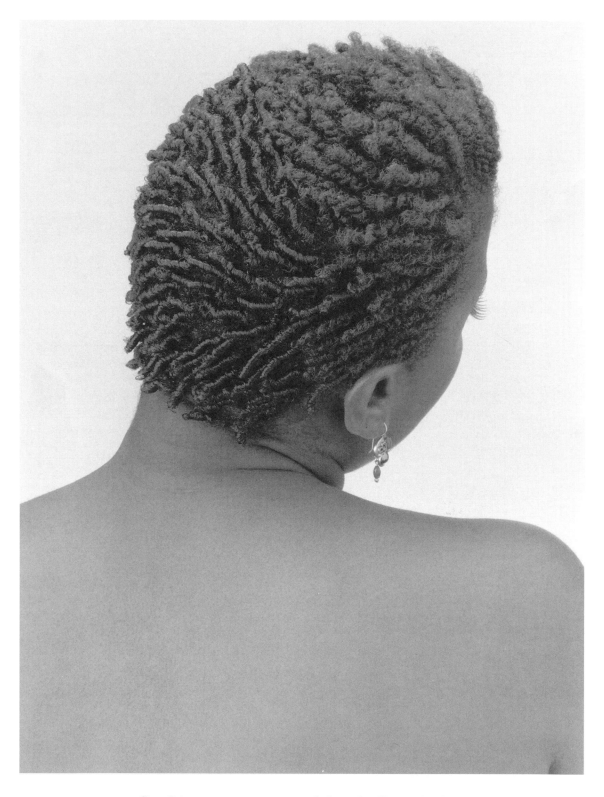

Combination wet twist with handrolls in the back.

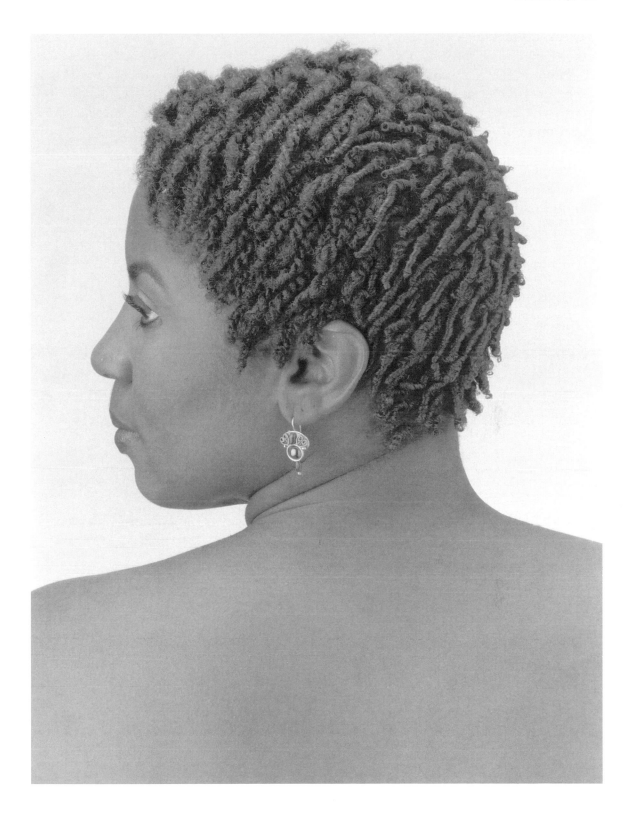

Textured hairline

A simple inverted braid or "roll" up the back can become more distinct with a textured hairline created using the twist knot wet set (pg. 124). This style works well if you don't have a lot of time but you want a style that is neat around the hairline edges and adds a touch of softness to the face.

1. **Part a 3-inch section along the entire hairline.**
2. **Moisten the fingertips with water and a small amount of gel, smooth on the hair and firmly rope twist along the hairline area.**
3. **Tie the hair flat for at least one hour or overnight.**
4. **Loosen out the hairline twist and blend the wavy hair into the roll, inverted braid or pinned up style.**

Blow dry & curl or press & curl

I do not recommend wearing this style frequently; however, if you feel the need to wear a straightened style, the blow dry and hot curl method makes this possible for natural hair. The combined heat from the blow dryer and curling iron will straighten the natural hair. Rather than trying to wear a straightened flat style, have the hair curled full to help reduce frizzing and swelling.

Always work on clean hair, use a light oil and hot curl small sections of hair at one time. Never apply heat to hair that is soiled or has hair spray, gel or mousse on it. In many cases hair is damaged due to very hot styling tools and soiled hair. For daily maintenance of a heat straightened style, use electric rollers rather than a hot curling iron. To maintain your curls, it is best to finger comb the hair. If your hair is naturally straight or wavy you can achieve a curled style with a wet set.

If you plan to wear natural styles like twist or handrolls, pressing or straightening the natural hair should be avoided. Heat straightening coily hair can stretch the hair, so that it does not coil back into its natural curl after wetting it. If your ends are straight and limp after wetting the hair, and the root is kinky, then you have heat damaged your hair and stretched out your natural curl. If you decide to wear twists or handrolls the straight, ends will have to be cut off.

For time's sake and best results, it is best to have your hair pressed or hot curled by a professional cosmetologist. Older beauticians are best skilled at this service; however, ask that they not use heavy grease, which makes the hair flat and stringy. As an alternative try twist-out texturing (pg.138) rather than heat straightening.

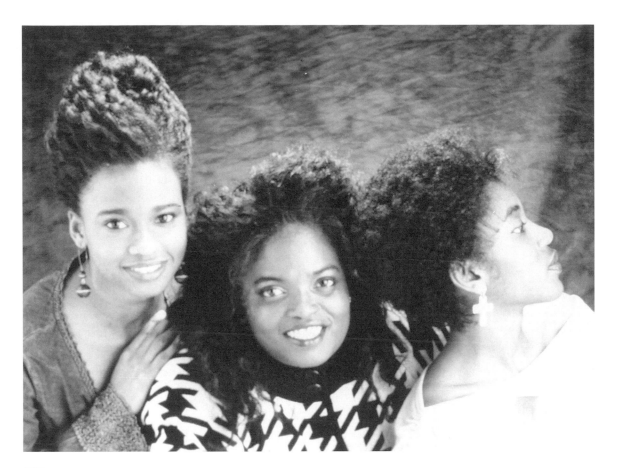

Twist out texturing

The twist technique can also be used to temporarily texture or wet set the hair. It is a way to enhance and set your natural curl depending on the method used. A thin or large twist would temporarily re-create the natural curl's size smaller or larger than it is. Like a wet set, once the hair is twisted, dampened and allowed to dry, a firm curl or crimp is set in the hair. The beauty of the twist-out is that you do not need grease and messy activators to maintain the curl. The natural nap in the hair and water are all you need.

Some women would contend that their hair is different and that "good hair" texture can only do this. Good hair is relative only to healthy hair; natural curl is based on texture. The individual twist-out style is beautiful on the curliest, nappiest and kinkiest hair textures; soft, wavy and straighter hair textures lack the strong curl needed to set a lasting natural twist out. Here are three ways to texture your hair in a twist out: individual twist out, flat twist wave, and with braids. Texturizing with these methods is temporary, same as a wet set or press and curl.

Individual twist out
1. Twist the hair the same as the individual twist. (see pg. 128)
2. Wet the hair thoroughly; apply a light natural gel or liquid hair oil to the edges and the twist ends. Smooth the edges, form the shape of the style and tie a scarf firmly on the hair to flatten it in place.
3. Allow the hair to dry completely, remove the scarf and untwist the hair. To untwist, put your finger between the two pieces of the twist and unwind the twist apart. This textured set will stay until the next shampoo. At bedtime cover the hair with a large scarf or Hair Tucker™; be sure to tie the hair in the direction you want the style to fall in. The next morning, hand paddle and restyle the hair in shape. To prevent the twist out style from frizzing, wear a plastic shower cap during hot baths or steamy showers.

Flat twist out wave
The flat twist out wave can be done with many tight flat twists or a few loose flat twists. The twist size and tension of the twist creates the varying different looks. A few loose twist, creates a large deep wave; many tight twist (up to 15 small sections) creates a small krimpy wave. The twist out can be worn hanging or in a pin-up style.

Pre-plan the style.
1. For loose wave; shampoo, then blow dry smooth. (For a tight krimpy wave, do not blow dry the hair.)
2. Part the hair in narrow sections for the flat twistrows.
3. Rub onto the hair, a light gel with moistened fingertips, as you firmly criss-cross and rope twist the hair flat. Keep fingers close to the scalp, as you twist, so that the twist lays flat and smooth.
4. After the twisted hair has completely dried, loosen the flat twists and thread fingers through to the scalp to finger rub out the parts. Style and shape the hair as you like.
5. At bedtime, cover with a large scarf or slumber cap.

Braid twist out
Same textured style as the twist out except individually braid or cornrow large braids while the hair is damp. After the hair has completely dried, unbraid, work fingers through the hair at the scalp and stretch the hair out to give it volume.

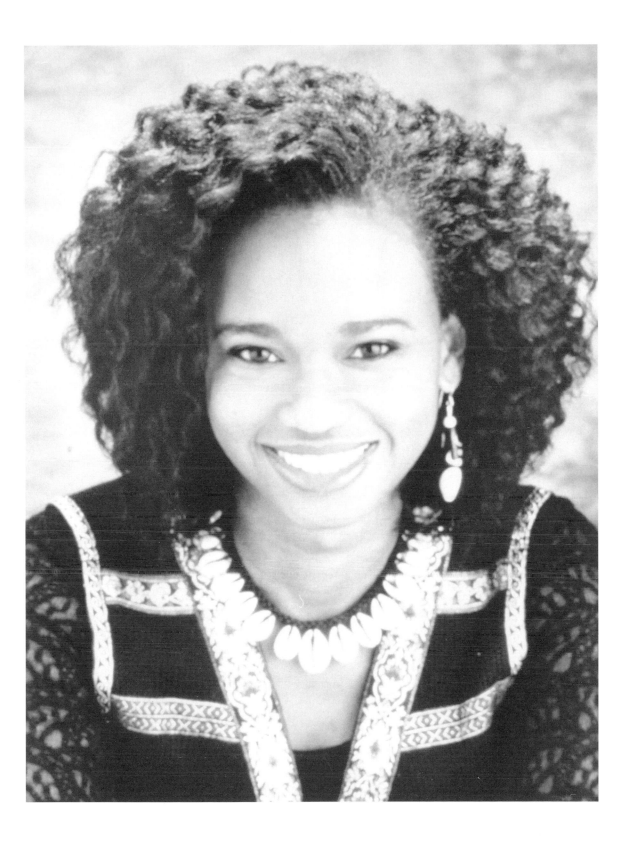

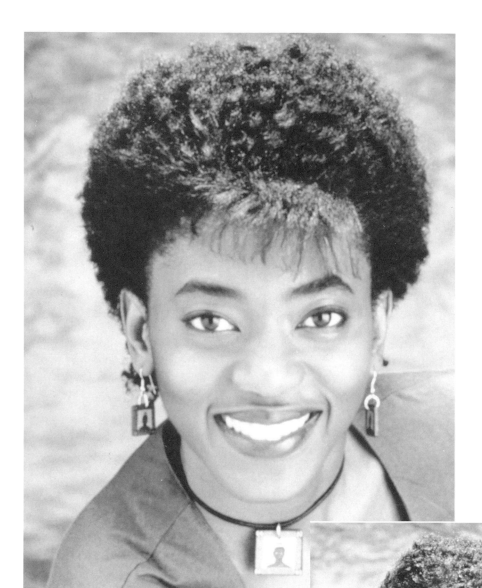

Small twistout wave

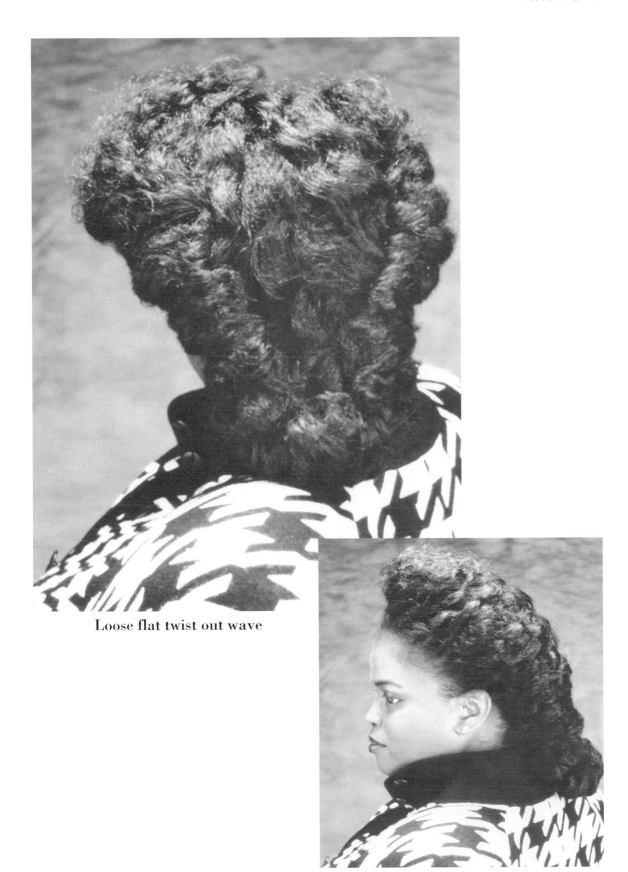

Loose flat twist out wave

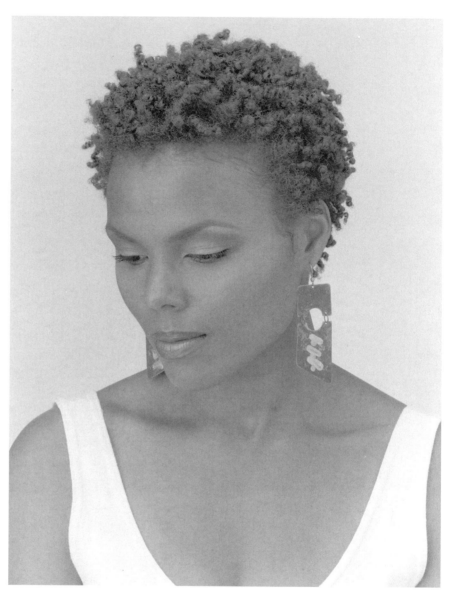

Individual twistout

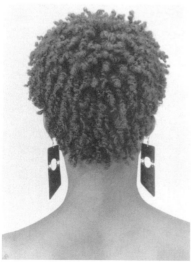

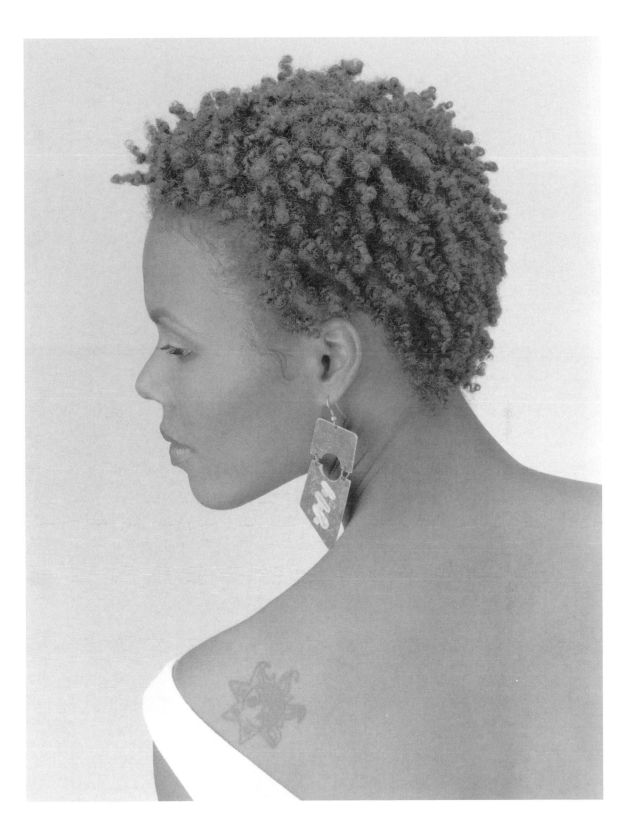

Do-it-yourself cornrows...

As a hair braider, I often assume all women can braid and cornrow. However, to my surprise, this is not the case. When I would suggest to clients to put a simple braid in their hair to hold them between salon visits, I found that they never learned to cornrow their own hair. And usually, women who know how to do an over hand braid don't know how to do an underhand braid, and vice-versa. This simple cornrow "how-to" is designed to help you learn the basic cornrow braid methods. This is not intended to teach you how to do hair extension styles, which should only be done by a professional hair braider.

One of the key elements to learning how to cornrow is practice. Don't expect to perfect this on the first try, or you will feel frustrated. Don't attempt your first try just before you have somewhere special to go. Experiment and practice in the mirror when you have time to take it out and retry as many times as possible.

A simple overhand cornrow, which is sometimes called a "French braid" (re-named by French settlers who colonized West Africa), will be referred to here as the African braid or overhand cornrow.

Using your hair ——
Underhand and Overhand Cornrow

1. Comb the hair together in the area where you want the braid.

2. Divide the top of the section into three equal pieces: left piece (1), middle piece (2), right piece (3).

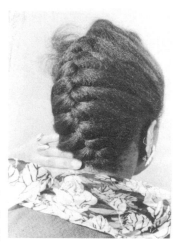

3. For the **invert overhand cornrow**, begin braiding by placing the left(1) or right(3) piece <u>over</u> the middle piece(2) and continue this alternately. As you are cornrow braiding along the narrow part, incorporate small pieces of hair from the outer side into the right and left piece as you place it <u>over</u> the middle piece. The inverted braid lays flat and smooth. (photo 1)

4. The **outward underhand cornrow** is braided the same way except the left(1) and right(2) pieces are placed <u>under</u> the middle piece(3) in an underhand motion creating a braid that is raised from the scalp. This braid slightly protrudes, giving it fullness. (photo 2)

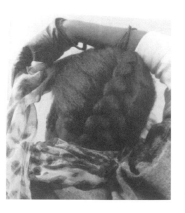

How to find a natural hair care stylist

There will come a time when your natural tresses need professional care. Hair braiders often are limited in braid techniques. Cosmetologists often are limited in working with straightened and chemical hair. So where do you find a natural hair care stylist? There is no easy answer, since this is a new field of practice. Finding a natural hair care stylist will depend on your ability to communicate to a braider, cosmetologist, or stylist about what your hair needs and expectations are. Once you know enough about your hair, you can set goals and objectives that the hair braider or stylist can work with.

You now know how to grow the chemical out of the hair, what style options are best suited for your hair condition, and the many styles that can be done to your natural texture. Remember, this is all new information, new methods that are not taught in beauty schools and a whole new approach to caring for the black woman's hair. Look for a hair braider who knows about hair care and is willing to try new styles without extensions. Some hair braiders do know how to do the natural styles discussed here, such as twists, natural texturing, and sculpted hair. Another option is to find a cosmetologist who has an affinity for cutting and styling and who does not favor chemicals. Share this book with them so they can learn to naturally care for your hair.

If you find a cosmetologist, start out by having conditioning treatments. This will give you an opportunity to know how the stylist handles your hair and feels about its curly kinky texture. If it is positive, then you have found a stylist you can work with; if the stylist tries to convince you to put a mild chemical in your hair run away pretty! Look for women who have natural hair like yours and a style you like. Ask who their stylist is. Check at cultural events, health spas, and naturopathic clinics for names of stylists who care for the hair naturally. In time, as more natural hair stylists are trained, there will be an abundance of naturalists providing healthy hair care services. If you have no luck finding a natural hair care stylist, do your own hair until you find one.

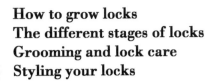

How to grow locks
The different stages of locks
Grooming and lock care
Styling your locks

Locking the hair is a part of good health because hair has more functions than beauty; it is one of the sensory parts of the body. Through it, we can feel tingles, shock, goose bumps, quivers and many other sensations. It holds the body's greatest amount of silicon, which is the "feeling and magnetic" element of the body. Your hair, therefore, is a receptor that helps to keep you magnetically balanced. The less it is handled and destroyed, the more sensitive and functional it will become.

Any style of unaltered, natural African hair symbolizes the very Africanness that many have come to misunderstand and dislike. The Masai men of Kenya, Bushmen of the Kalahari, Africa; Rastafarians, and African people around the world wear locks. There is nothing new about it, except that more and more African Americans have chosen this style and wear it for many reasons. The new resurgence of "Black Pride" has made locks a popular style worn for various reasons including spiritual, cultural, fashion and health.

I will refer to this hair style as "locks" or "hair locks," a name that is endearing, fitting and in line with it's true spirit. There's nothing dreadful about locks so to refer to locked hair as "dreads" continues to perpetuate the negative, mean-spirited contempt for this natural hair. Any hair that is unclean, nasty and unkempt, whether it is straight, blonde, permed, relaxed or natural, is dreadful.

The popularity of locks has created a new service in the hair care industry. Hair stylists who once frowned upon nappy textured hair must now learn about a natural style that supersedes all previously learned European hair styling methods done in the modern salon. As salons and the general public come to appreciate this style as another dimension of hair, the negative stereotypes and false images many associate with it will fade.

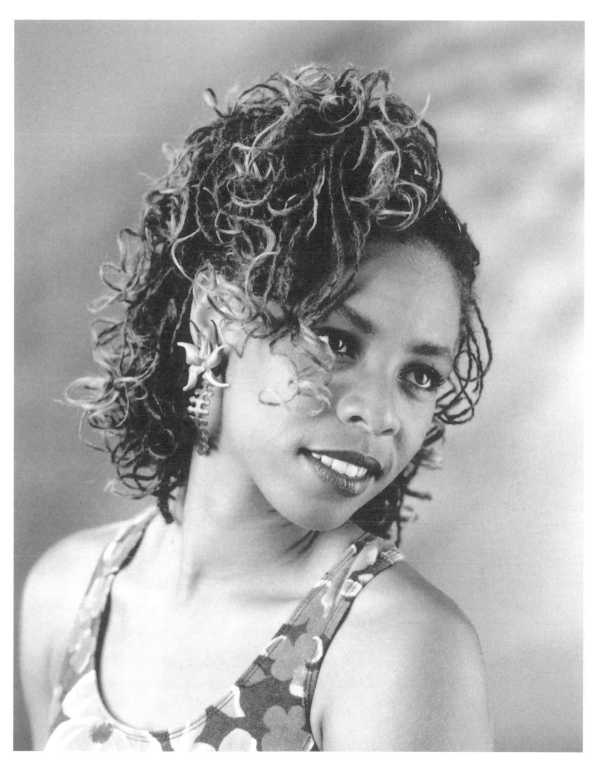

Photo Courtesy Sisterlocks®

Unfortunately though, people who wear their hair in the style of locks confront unreasonable, disdain even within their own race. They are unfairly judged, discriminated against and treated differently. Fear and ignorance cause people to view locks as unsanitary, unkempt, radical and from another culture. The idea that one would wear the hair uncombed and in a non-European style, to them, is threatening; to say the least. Educated black folks were raised to pride themselves on the quality and texture of their straightened hair. Hair that was not straight, and surely not combed, was considered an embarrassment and a disgrace.

It is not unusual for the black family to disown a relative for wearing uncombed locked hair. One client tells of how she is banned from her parent's house because of her locks. I heard another sad incident from one of my clients from Cameroon, Africa. She is a student in Washington, DC, who has come to the salon for over a year to have her nu-locks groomed and styled. We painstakingly worked to get her locks to grow long and uniform. One day she called the salon wanting to know what we could do to her hair to remove or change the locks because she was going home to visit her family.

Well, mind you, locks are quite permanent and cannot be transformed into unlocked hair without cutting them off. Her locks had grown out really beautifully and the style was fantastic on her. I sensed she did not really want to get rid of her locks but she said she had to, because she could not go home with her hair like this. Her family and the people within her village would think she was mentally ill. She said, "They feel only a crazy person would wear her hair like that." I suggested that she cover it with beautiful head wraps and educate them about this hair style. She had such anguish, cutting off her locks was the only way she felt she could visit her family. She feared the rejection and retaliation from her family and friends if she wore her hair in that style "back home." This fear is a reality for black people around the world.

Our community is open to many forms of cultural and artistic expression; however, hair worn in an African inspired style does not meet this same openness. Because of differences, people sometimes build up fears and create hateful labels that alienate people of their own race. Some would suggest this is how the terms "dreadlocks, dreads, or knotty dread" came to be. Uncombed hair was viewed as dreadful. It is an appropriate name when you think about how established society dreads the hair texture of the black man and woman. In fact if you were to look up the definition of the word dread, it means *to fear greatly; frightening, extremely distasteful, unpleasant, and shocking.*

To further compound the misunderstanding of locks, for years, anyone who locked their hair was referred to as a Rastafarian. If you wore locks you were from Jamaica and of the Rastafarian community. The visibility of Jamaican artists, such as Bob Marley, exposed more Americans to locked hair. All people who wear locks are obviously, not Jamaican; all Jamaican's are not Rastafarian, and all Rastafarians are not from Jamaica.

The Rastafarian beginnings were not in Jamaica, but in Africa. The first Rastafarians appeared in Jamaica in 1930, at the time of Ras Tafari's coronation as Emperor Haile Selassie of Ethiopia[11]. Rastafari is a culture that is now prevalent in Jamaica, but has its strong religious and philosophical roots in Africa. It is a peaceful, spiritual, and African centered way of life, a culture that is diverse and complex in its philosophies and practices.

It is important to talk about the Rastafarian community and their way of life to clear up misconceptions and fears people may have developed. Rastafarians in Jamaica were considered a sub-class or sub-culture by blacks under colonial rule. The European-educated, black Jamaican's, were taught to fear and hate the Rastafarian, whose life is everything reminiscent of the African heritage. The Rastafarian diet, language, dress, spiritual beliefs and hair style all became constant reminders. Many Rastafarian men will cover their locks with a wool tam of the adopted African Liberation colors; red, black, and green (with gold) before going out in public. For religious reasons, and out of respect for their cultural heritage, Rastafarian women cover their hair in public.

Some American "black nationalist" wear locks as a political statement; "their right to be themselves." Their locks are sacred to them, so much so, that they don't believe in having anyone else groom or handle them. I can remember some years ago, these nationalists and others were wary of a salon advertisement for grooming locks. Now, however, a new population is wearing locks -- doctors, lawyers, housewives, children and even cosmetologists. Yes, there are cosmetologists who wear locks but perm their clients hair. Such a contradiction for a naturalist!

Style is mostly what many lock wearers want today. For them, locks have nothing to do with natural living, and nothing to do with a political or cultural statement; but everything to do with preferred style. This style is so individualistic and cooperative with the natural curl in black people's hair. Keep in mind, many of the new lock wearers are people who previously permed, relaxed, pressed, weaved and "fixed" their hair. Many have said they were tired of fighting their hair texture and wanted a hair style that was really permanent, however they still want salon care. The braid salon, locktician, natural stylist and even chemical-toting cosmetologist see benefit in salon care for locks. Straightening the hair is no longer a subject of discussion in the salon for the lock wearer.

Clients who come to the salon for locks often say they want to lock their hair for low maintenance, individual style, or because it is a fad. Recently, a young oriental boy came into the salon with his dad for a consultation to have his hair locked like the hair style he saw on the young members of a hip hop singing group. I had to explain that the hair had to grow into the style over a period of time and that it was not possible to get "true locks" in a one-day styling session at the salon. Many people think locked hair is created at the salon, not realizing the hair must grow into the style. Because the hair style requires commitment and time, locks as a fad is contrary to reason. Fads come and go, are impulsive and are generally founded on making quick money. Although imitation locks are impressive, the high cost to do them and long time it takes is prohibitive for the "fad lock wearer."

Regardless of the reasons people want locks, one thing is clear; lock wearers want information and service to care for their hair naturally "sans extensions." I believe more people would wear the lock style if they had support from family, friends and salons that specialize in the care and grooming of locks. Every head of hair is different and may require a variance for growing the locks. People need sensible, safe hair care information. I've heard inquiries such as, "Do you wash them?" "Are they dirty?" "Should I use bees wax?" "Will clay make the hair lock?" "Can I have them done in a day?" and "Can I comb them out when I am tired of them?" Until recently, there have been no tried and tested standards for basic lock grooming and hair care. This chapter will give a step-by-step approach on how you can grow a luxurious head of beautiful healthy locks. It is the result of years of work guiding clients through the different phases of preparing and caring for their hair locks. Even though the hair will lock differently on each person's hair type, the basic beginning process, grooming instruction, and care regimen are the same.

HOW TO GROW LOCKS

Wearing locks is a long time commitment. It is the closest you will get to a "hair permanent," since the hair form is unchangeable. Locks are formed when uncombed hair tangles and mats into clusters. These clusters can be formed small or very thick, depending on how you decide to start your locks. When the hair starts to actually mat and lock together, there is no turning back; the hair cannot be combed out or loosened apart. So this is a style that takes pre-planning, patience and devotion. Once you have decided this is for you, there is a reality factor that it does not happen overnight, in a week or even a month. At some stages in the growing process you may not like your hair, especially if your goal is to have long locks. The long, beautiful, shoulder-length locks you have seen on someone else probably took up to four years to grow. Unless you are willing to make a long-term commitment to this style, skip this chapter and go to the individual braid or twist style section of the book. If you are willing to take the time to grow locks, then continue reading to find out what you can expect during this long dedicated process.

You can form your hair into locks in two ways, the *free-form* or the *guided form*.
"Free form" locks are grown by simply shampooing the hair and allowing it to grow without ever combing, twisting, shaping or brushing. The hair naturally grows in irregular clusters with no uniformity. One free-form way that is done in Africa is to towel dry short hair in circular motions so that the hair freely forms in tightly separated curls.
With the "guided form," you pre-determine the shape of the locks with twists, braids or handrolls. This style, also referred to as "salon locks," is sectioned and stylized into

neat, uniform locks. They are trained to grow in a particular size and shape. Salon locks require the most care and attention. If you are looking for a no maintenance hair style, the free-from is recommended over the guided form. Contrary to popular belief, "salon locks," especially, are not care-free. This style requires regular grooming, re-twisting and new growth separation if the hair is to look fresh and neat at the scalp. In fact, there is no hair style that is truly care-free; all hair requires regular cleansing and grooming. Even a bald head needs to be shaved, unless the hair loss is permanent.

Since free-form locks do not need to be separated and re-twisted at the new growth, these locks are considered low maintenance. <u>Low</u> maintenance should not be confused with <u>no</u> maintenance. Free-form locks need shampooing, conditioning and scalp care. Guided salon locks, on the other hand, require re-twisting of the new hair growth regularly and some grooming attention.

Here are several different ways to begin locking your hair:
Free-form, Two-strand twist, Braids, Handrolls, Beading,, Wrapping, Sisterlocks®

Free-Form
In this process you will let the natural hair grow in the shape, size and form that nature sees fit. The locks will not be uniform and the shape and size will grow irregular. Some may grow as thin as pencils, others may grow as large as your wrist.

1. Shampoo the natural hair with a degreasing non-moistruizing shampoo.

2. After rinsing thoroughly, towel dry the excess water, ruffle and rub the hair in circular motions with a towel to give the uncombed Afro some definition and separation (works best on short length hair).

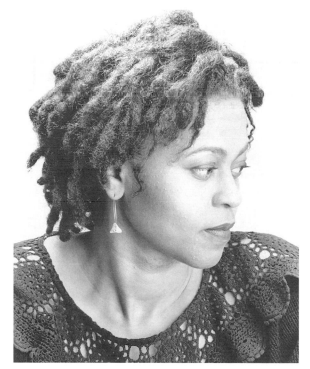

3. Allow the hair to air dry. Never comb the hair again. Repeat this process each time the hair is wet or shampooed. (Towel rub the hair in the same direction each time.)

Continue to care for the hair like this and eventually the hair will mold and form into locks. Coarser, thicker curly hair will mat and group faster than soft, wavy, straight texture hair. Every day, wet the hair to swell and re-shape areas that have flattened from sleeping on it. It could take up to six months for the hair to start to mat and form locks of hair.

Two-strand twist for locking

This process gives the hair a soft puffy appearance that resembles locks. The kink and small tight curl in African-American hair helps it to easily form locks.

The size and tension of the twist will determine the size of the lock. For a small lock, twist the hair tightly. To prevent locks from breaking off at the new growth as they get long and heavy, section the hair in pencil size twists. If the twists are too small or thin, the locks are prone to break off as they grow longer. The thin base cannot hold the weight of the lengthy lock. This is all a part of pre-planning the correct size of sections to start your locks. Clients who have started their locks with too small sections come to the salon to try and save the locks that are dangling, long and heavy, on a thin base of hair. Once you have invested the time to grow your locks long, the last thing you want to contend with is the possibility of them breaking off. Another way to prevent breakage is to always re-twist the new growth hair in the same direction. Handroll the new growth hair in the same direction (left or right) each time so that you never forget the direction you train your locks.

If you want to grow fine micro locks there is a method called *Sisterlocks $_{Tm}$* that guides the hair in small locks that are lightweight even as the locks grow long. This style of locks duplicates the styling flexibility and movement of loose hair. The initial process is intricate and can take up to 12 hours. This technique must be done by a skilled practitioner.

It is important to make the right size section for your hair texture so that you will be happy with your locks after years of growing. To have to re-size locks after the hair has begun to lock would involve starting over or creating fork-like locks. Doubling the new growth hair of two locks creates a fork end that has two locks.

To begin locks with the two-strand twist does not work well for all hair textures and conditions. If the hair is freshly cut, soft, wavy, straight or less that five inches, the twist will unravel and need to be re-twisted often during the beginning months. Soft, deep wavy, or large curl hair does not lock well because the large curl in the natural hair will not stay tightly together. The two-strand twist is dependent on the small curl that tightly binds the hair together. Although the two-strand twist method gives an almost immediate appearance of locked hair, it also requires immediate grooming.

How-to start locks with twist

1. Section the hair into the desired size for the locks, (not too small.)

2. Divide the hair into two even pieces and criss-cross the two pieces of hair to form a rope texture. Twist in the same direction throughout the head. The kink and curl in the hair is what holds the twist ends together.

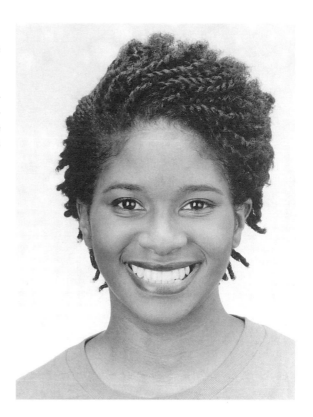

Individual braid for locking

Starting locks with a braid is the last resort for the impatient one, whose hair is not ready to stay together on its own.

Locks that are started with braids grow out with the braid on the ends. Even after many years of growing, the braid never changes. So you may have six inches of locked hair with a two-inch braid at the end. Of course you can always cut off the braid once the hair is formed with some length. The individual braid method is a three-strand plait. Even though small braids are attractive, if the sections are too small, the locked hair may break off easily at the new growth due to improper handling. Section the hair in pencil size

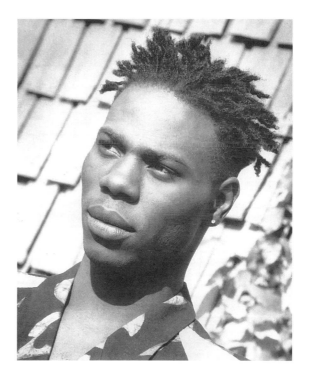

How-to start locks with braids:

1. Starting at the nape, section the hair in a pencil size diameter.

2. Divide the section into three pieces and braid to the very end of the hair. Each braid should be the same size with loose tension (if possible).

thickness to be sure the base hair can withstand the maintenance handling. The braid lock method is quite durable and has the appearance of being flat and smaller compared to the twist. Shampoo the hair as normal, letting it air dry. Leave the hair braided until the new growth starts to mat and form hair locks. The braid may hold better for hair that is short and soft because the three stitches secure the hair ends together.

Maintenance for braid locks is different since the braid is not puffy and is less likely to unravel and loosen at the base. The new growth of the braid is contained because the braid does not unwind at the scalp area; the new growth of the twist slightly unwinds making the re-twisting process more frequent than the braid. This difference is minor unless the hair length and texture are not suitable for the soft twist. If the hair type is suitable for both the braid and the twist, the choice between the two should be twist.

The braid with extension is another last resort alternative to lock hair that is damaged, extremely short, blunt ends and not in the best condition to grow locks naturally. With the help of extensions, the hair can be braided or twisted and left to grow out long enough to start locking on its own. Once the lock is at least three inches or more you may cut off the extension braid. This process must be done by a skilled hair braider. Many clients who have chemically treated hair choose this option.

Sisterlocks®

This system was designed by Dr. Jo-Anne Cornwell for creating fine, micro locks. It must be done by a trained practitioner. The Sisterlock® is created by a backward braid technique that interweaves strands of hair into a permanent lock of hair. This method can also be used on some permed hair.

Handrolls for locks

The hair is literally rolled into a coil. The size handroll is determined by the size curl in the hair and the section. The tighter and smaller the curl, the shorter and narrower the handroll. A loose wave hair texture does not hand roll well because the curl is not small enough to firmly hold together.

Although handrolls are not the quickest way to begin locks, it is another option and is chosen mostly for style. Locks set from the handrolls take a long while for the hair to begin locking. This type of lock actually is worn for style more than lock-ability. Smooth, shiny and tube shaped, it looks like a cultivated salon lock. The lock is unique and exotic, giving the hair a glazed polish effect when a natural gel is used. This style is called the handroll because the curl is actually created using the hands in a rolling motion from the base to the ends. Because the hair end usually is not secure, when the hand roll is shampooed it will uncoil.

Re-rolling the hair is a continuous and ongoing process and it can take eight months before the handrolls become trained to stay in the hair after a shampoo. The frequent salon visits to re-roll can make this a costly style, and more difficult to do on yourself than the twist or braids. Handrolls are best if you want to start small locks. The stylish look, for some, is worth more than it costs.

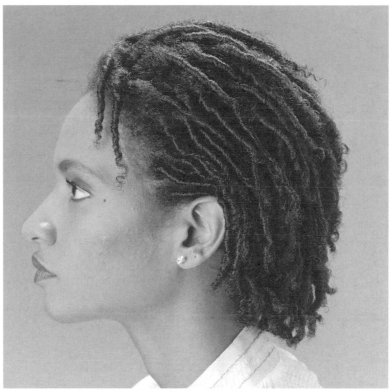

Handrolls to start locks.

Beading and Thread wrapping

An ornate and artsy way to lock the hair is to slide beads onto sections of hair or wrap the entire length of hair with thread. Select beads or thread that you will want to wear everyday until the new growth hair forms locks. Once the hair forms locks and grows long, the beads will be at the lock ends. You can eventually cut off the beaded portion of hair or, if possible, slide the beads off to keep the full length of the hair. For thread wrapped hair simply remove the thread from the locked hair.

How long does it take the hair to lock?

I have had many clients come to the salon asking for locks as if they can be created in a day. Most people cannot imagine a hair style that takes years to form. The beauty industry thrives on fast changing styles that are fashioned in a salon visit. And there have been imitation styles to try and introduce locks as another "fast" style. Although the imitation locks (silky lock method) do not take years to form, they can take up to 12 hours or more to do. There is nothing like genuine locks that are grown with time and love -- a process that can take months and years to grow. Depending on the softness, coarseness, size of your natural curl or kink, your hair may lock quickly in weeks or take months. Coarse, curly, kinky hair locks the fastest. Coarse hair, which is considered suitable locking hair, on an average, will begin to form locks in two to four months. This hair type can be shampooed more frequently and conditioned for sheen.

Soft, wavy or straighter hair takes twice as long to lock. This hair texture can take up to one year to begin matting. The reason a soft, straight texture takes a longer time to lock is that the hair softens during shampooing which impedes tangling and matting. One way to keep the hair from softening is to not condition it after a shampoo, since the conditioner coats and separates the hair strands. Avoid using conditioning and moisture rich shampoos. Instead use a striping or degreasing shampoo. The objective is to roughen the hairs cuticle, causing it to mat together.

THE STAGES OF LOCKING

The locking process has three stages: *beginning, intermediate and rooted.*
It is important to become familiar with the three stages so that you know what to do, what to look for, and what to expect of your hair while it is growing and forming locks.

Beginning Stage (first 6 months)
The beginning stage, also called baby locks, is when the hair is not quite locked yet. From inception to forming shape, this is when the hair is most delicate and requires special handling and nourishment. It is the process of grouping the hair to form the pre-determined size locks. At this phase the hair is only assembled and may give a stylized appearance of locked hair. Based on the length and texture of the hair, in some cases the initial lock may appear sparse and crude. Thin hair may show scalp, while thicker, coarser hair will look fashionable from the beginning. This, too, will depend on how well you work with your hair by shaping and sculpting it into a style during this "rough sketch" period. Grooming and embellishing the hair with head wraps helps with style when the locks are too short to lay neat.

At this phase of beginning locks, style is essential; however, the more important thing is to start the hair with the right size sections so the locks will grow strong and supported, and it is important to keep the scalp and hair clean for good hygiene.

Intermediate Stage (12-18 months)
The intermediate stage is the period of growth between the baby locks and the mature rooted locks. I like to call it the adolescent period for locks. The locked hair will develop and grow, taking on a life of its own. You will really have to be watchful and a consistent guide to cultivate the hair into well made locks. It is a crucial phase because it

determines how well the locks will grow and how beautifully they form. During this phase, the hair will go through a series of changes. In some instances it will do things you do not want it to do. You can expect the hair to frizz, unravel at the edges, and even seem unkempt. Do not worry; the natural hair is simply taking shape and form. As you continue to groom and guide the locks, the new growth hair should begin to form and take hold rather than growing out as a bush or Afro under the locking ends.

Once new growth begins to bush, you will need to separate and re-twist this new hair. Separating and twisting the new hair, regularly, will keep your locks looking fresh, neat and well groomed. Such locks will give the effect of uniform, individual braids. The intermediate stage is also a time of adjusting and getting comfortable with a look that is transforming before your eyes.

Don't be surprised or bothered by unsolicited remarks about your hair from people around you. You can expect ignorant comments and obvious discomfort from family, co-workers and the public. Don't be surprised by those who try to control your hair and your decision to lock. If you are prepared for this, it will not make you feel insecure and second guess your brave decision. For silly remarks, simply reply "I love my hair, so should you." And then if you are up to it, try to educate those who question your natural hair.

Rooted stage (2 years or more)

The most respected locks are the ones that are rooted. They are a mark of honor showing your commitment, devotion and comfort with your hair. The term "rooted" means they are formed, shaped and settled into their decided style. You are truly at the point of no return, no comb-out and no loosening the hair apart. The locks have become established into their shape and size. At this point you should set a regular schedule to manage and re-twist the new growth hair as the locks grow long. On an average, locks that are five years old are below shoulder length; and 10-year-old locks can grow to waist length. Although this phase is rooted, there can be growing problems that need special attention and care.

As the locks become long and too heavy on certain areas of the hair, they may cause discomfort. Another common problem for the mature locks is thinning at the scalps base, causing the locks to break off. This happens if the locks were started using too small a section of hair and the heavy weight of the long locks dangling weakens the base hair. Age, wear and tear of shampooing, health problems that affect the hair, and styling can also cause the locks to weaken.

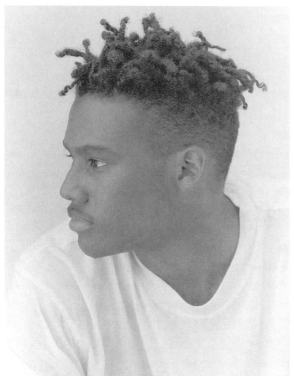

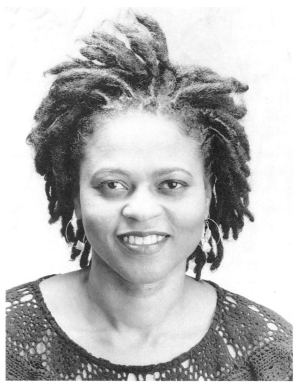

Beginning stage 3 mos.
Started with individual twist

Intermediate stage 10 mos.
Started by free-form

Rooted stage
10 years

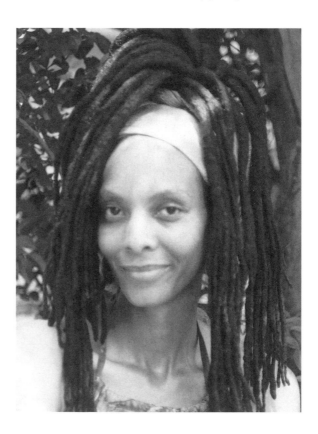

Grooming and Lock Care

When you look around and see so many people wearing locks; the size, texture, color, length and quality of each person's hair is what makes their locks unique. Some locks are well groomed, cultivated, stylized and fashionable; then, there are what I would classify as unrefined natural locks; the ones that are unhandled, uncultivated, so that the hair grows naturally into its own original and beautiful unmatched form. However, style has nothing to do with cleanliness. I have seen unkempt locks; the ones that are not regularly shampooed or groomed, making the hair look dull, dry and raggedy. Unfortunately, these raggedy locks can give all lock wearers a bad name.

As the saying goes, "Cleanliness is next to Godliness." Whether natural, permed or locked, clean hair is essential. Unfortunately one of the myths about locks is that the hair is unclean. There are unqualified stylists or novice lock wearers who believe that they should not shampoo their hair for months in order for the hair to begin to lock. First-time clients come to the salon with their hair in handrolls or twists and have not shampooed their hair in months because whoever (friend, hair stylist, braider) put the style in also instructed them that water would loosen their hair and prevent it from locking. This is incorrect and absolutely absurd. All hair should be shampooed regularly, so that it does not become a breeding place for bacteria and germs. If a hair stylist instructs you not to shampoo your hair for extended periods of time, this is a sure sign that this stylist is not familiar with the hair locking process.

In many cases, I've seen hair that was too short, evenly cut, very soft and not suitable to begin locks. It is important to understand your hairs condition and what method will allow you to keep your hair and scalp clean while growing locks. If the hair does not hold a twist, braid or handroll (for whatever reason), you must wait until the hair is in the condition to do so or add extensions to hold the hair together. If you start with bad grooming habits, you will more than likely continue this as the hair forms locks. I'm sure we would all agree that unkempt, dirty locks give all locks a bad name. Seeing raggedy locks perpetuates the idea that people who wear locks do not shampoo their hair. So with basic grooming tips, establish a hair care regimen that allows you the time to regularly shampoo and style your locks.

Even though there is no need for combing and brushing, well groomed locks require a lot of time and care. Beautiful locks are regularly shampooed, conditioned, oiled, separated and re-twisted as the hair grows out.

Shampoo and grooming

I recommend that you shampoo your locks as often as needed. Once a week or every two weeks is normal; however, depending on your personal need, you may shampoo more frequently.

To shampoo beginner locks:
1. Rinse the hair thoroughly in the shower.
2. Mix a mild (non-conditioning) natural shampoo with with a little water into a lather in the hands and gently massage the lathered shampoo onto the scalp and then squeeze it through the twists or braids. Handrolls will require delicate massaging and even this does not ensure that the handrolls will not unwind.
3. Rinse the shampoo from the hair.
4. Apply conditioner rinse to the scalp and the hair ends; leave on for five minutes, then rinse thoroughly and towel dry the hair to remove the excess water. *(If the beginner locks are short or the hair is soft, do not apply conditioner; as this may soften the hair more, causing it to unravel.)*
5. For a sheen, rub a dime sized amount of liquid oil in the hands and work it through to the hair ends. To smooth and flatten frizzy edges, tie the hair with a cotton scarf or Hair Tucker" while the hair is still wet; leave the hair tied until it is dry. Remove the scarf and the edges will look neat and flat. This is also a way to shape and direct the style. For example, if you like the hair off the face, tie the hair back or for a Cleopatra effect, tie the hair downward.

To shampoo intermediate locks:
1. Wet the hair thoroughly in the shower then work lathered shampoo onto the scalp and squeeze it out to the locked ends.
2. Rinse the shampoo out of the hair and apply conditioner rinse to the scalp and the lock ends; leave on for five minutes; then rinse thoroughly and towel dry the hair to remove the excess water
3. For a sheen on the hair, (follow step 5. above)
4. To separate the new growth hair, gently pull apart and palm roll each lock , concentrating on the loose scalp hair. Separate and palm roll the new growth hair every three to four weeks.

To shampoo rooted locks
Shampoo the hair the same as you would the intermediate locks, except you must work the lather into three to four locks at a time, depending on the thickness and length. Thick, long locks may take several hours or a full day to completely air dry. During summer months or in year-round hot climates, it is best to let the hair dry naturally. For colder climates, plan to shampoo your hair on a day you do not need to leave the house or dry the hair with an electric dryer.

STYLING YOUR LOCKS

Lock styles are only limited by your imagination. Explore the many styling possibilities that can be done to your locks. The thinner and longer the locks the more styling versatility you will have. Once the hair has some length to it, the feel and pliability is similar to braids. Some locks are very soft and pliable and other locks may be stiff and hard to bend or fold. This is where pre-planning is important. If you want thick locks you will be limited to hanging styles. For a variety of styling options, plan to grow thin, narrow locks. Of course soft locks give hair the most style options such as waving, wet set, sculpting, style cut, beaded and whatever else comes to mind. Some people are even coloring their locks; however, I caution against strong dye and chemical colors if natural is your forte.

Soft Locks
The feel and bendability of your locks depends on their size and what you put on the hair. Keep in mind, locks are hair. Many lock wearers pile so much "gook" and stuff on their locks, they can become hard. Certain products, pomades and gels do not easily rinse from the hair. Bees wax, clay, gels, heavy grease, spray and pink lotions all create a heavy build-up of residue that coats the hair, making it dull, grayish and stiff. Clean hair is light, soft, and lustrous.

Wavy Locks
Dampen the hair or immediately after a shampoo apply a light liquid oil and braid three to six locks together. Do this throughout the entire head. Allow the braided locks to dry naturally or under a hair dryer. Unbraid the locks and the hair has a strong wave texture that will last up to a week.

Wet Set
This is done exactly as a roller set on loose hair. The size and style roller (sponge, hard, spiral, perm rods) will determine the type of curl. A very large roller will create a full body effect; for above shoulder length locks it will give the locks a "Cleopatra" bend. Small rollers create a curly, spiral effect. Experiment with different types of curls. Another fun wet set style comes from winding the locks into a pin curl and securing with clips, then loosen once the hair is dry. For any of the wet set styles, first, dampen the hair or 30 minutes after a shampoo, apply a light liquid oil, then set the locks in groups of two to three throughout the entire head. Dry the roller set locks naturally or sit under a hair dryer for a quick dry.

Sculpted Locks
Locks that are pliable can be manipulated and styled into many hair designs. For the office, you can style the locks into contemporary rolls, beehives, and chignons. Any pin-up style that can be done with braids or loose hair is possible with locks. It takes practice, the right pins and just simply doing it.

To create an African roll for a contemporary conservative style, pull the hair together to a center point where you want the roll. Pin one side flat and roll the other side inward, gently tucking the ends into the roll. Pin the roll in position.

Pull the hair back into a bun, by gathering the locks secure with a fabric band. If the ends are long enough, tuck them around the band to cover and form a neat bun. If the locks are short, put a fine net over the ends to mold the locks into a rounded shape.

Lock Cut

For a dramatic, contemporary look, cut the locks into a precision style. Taper the back and sides, and cut the locks to chin length. For a layered, shag effect, cut the top shorter than the back. This style will keep length while cutting off some of the bulk around the face. If your locks appear thin, an even trim will give the illusion of fullness.

Beads and Colorful Wrapping

For embellishment you can give your locks a dressed up jeweled style. Embellishing and adding ornaments to the hair can be beautiful as well as functional. You can sew seed beads onto the locks or use a hairpin to place pearl size beads through the hair. Add beads, shells and trinkets to give your locks a creative edge. Select a bead with a hole that is large enough to slide up and position on the lock so that it does not slide off. For tiny beads and cowry shells, use a thin needle and thread to sew onto the lock. To add color or firm texture to locks, thread wrapping is popular. You can add silk thread, glitter or textured thread that resembles hair.

Pompadour Roll with Height.

Pull all the locks upward, fold the ends within the pompadour roll and pin the hair in place using large hair pins.

Sisterlocks®

Locks created by this process gives bounce, body, easy styling and an immediate style of locked hair. The Sisterlocks® system helps the hair to form fine tiny locks by using a special tool that utilizes your own natural hair to weave a sort of backward braid. Once the process is done, it is permanent and will not unravel easily. Because the locks are extremely thin they can be easily styled with rollers, curling irons and sculpted into contemporary or elegant up styles.

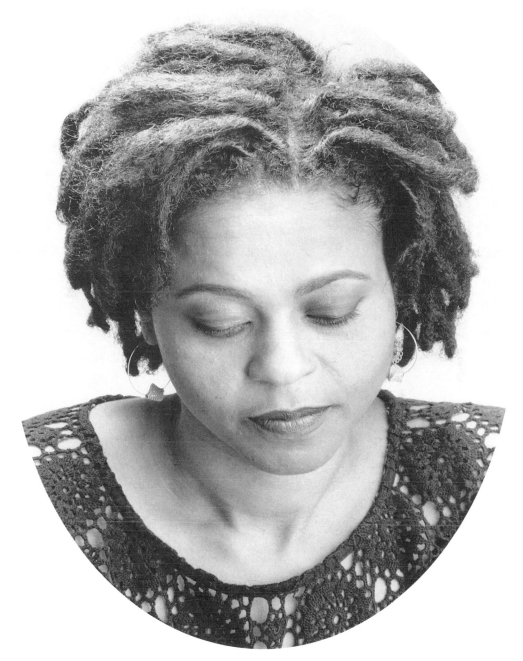

Locs-A-Body

A client shared with me a real simple way to give locks body.

1. Pull the locks up in a loose ponytail at the top of the head before entering the shower. (Do not wet the locks, let the steam and mist from the shower moisten the hair.)

2. Allow the moistened hair to thoroughly dry. Remove the ponytail and the hair will bob in a soft, full bodied, rounded shape.

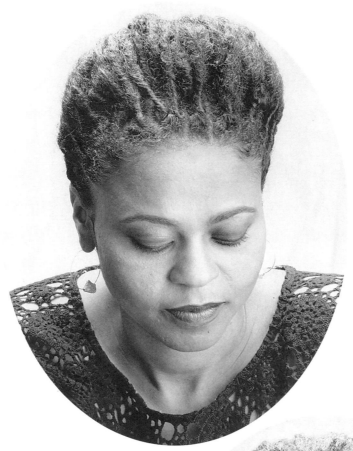

Pin-up locks

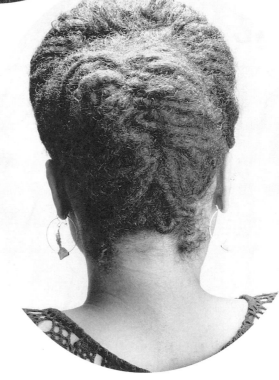

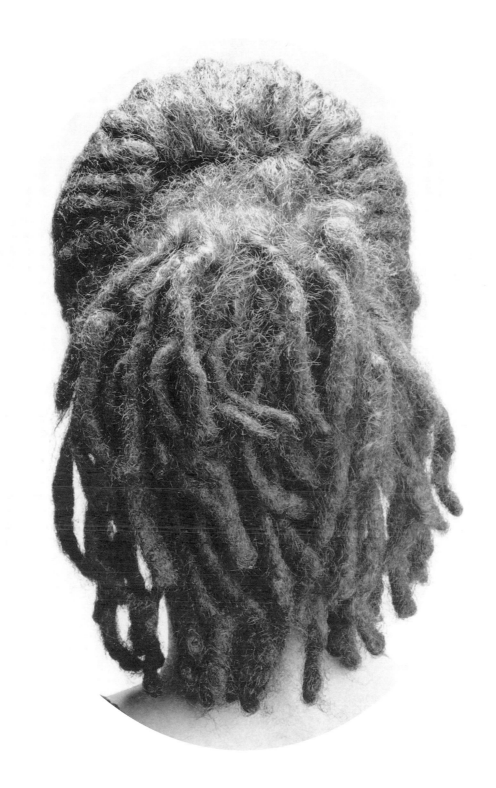

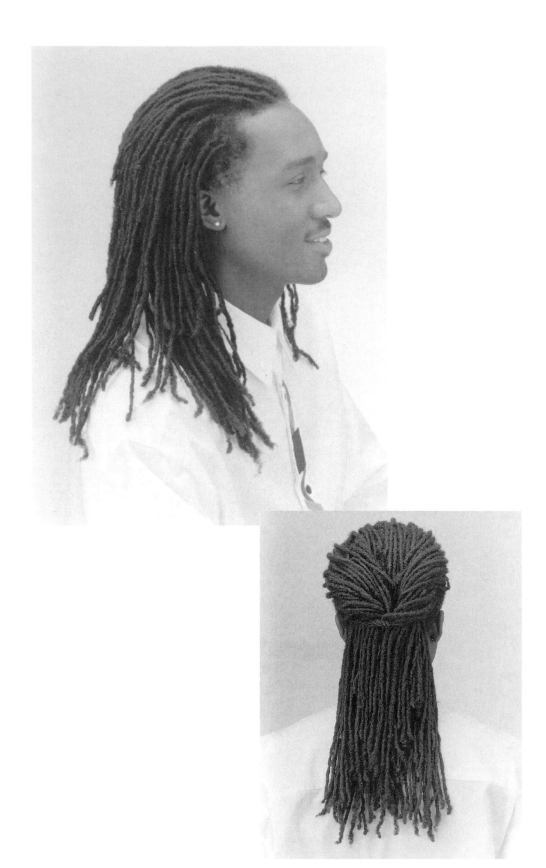

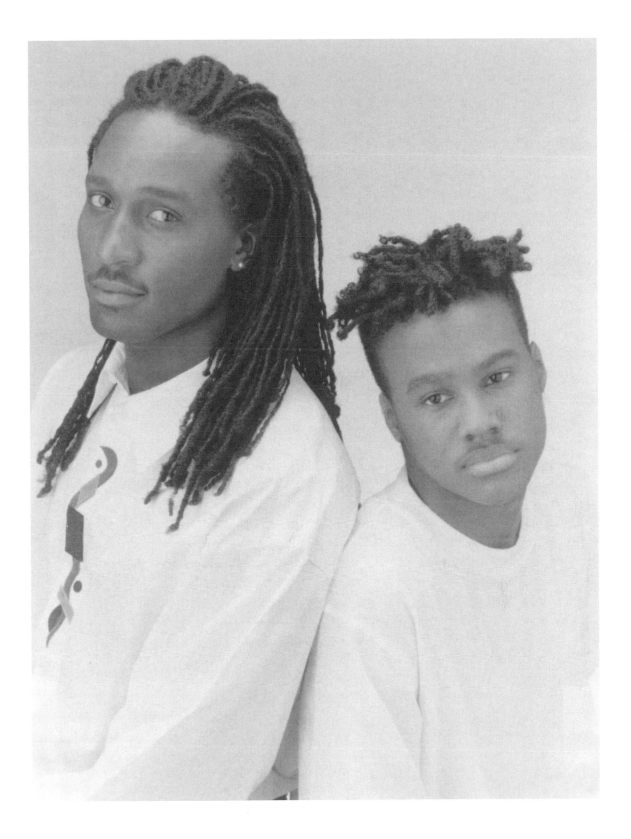

Sisterlocks® — *micro fine locks, curled and styled.*

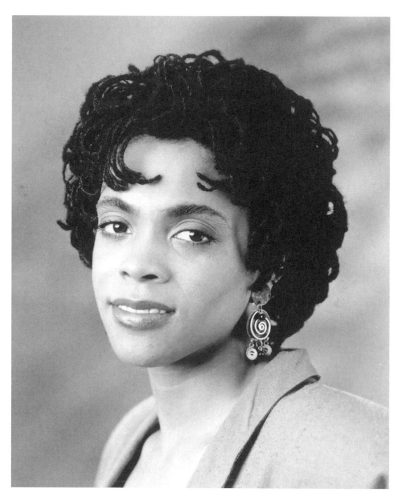

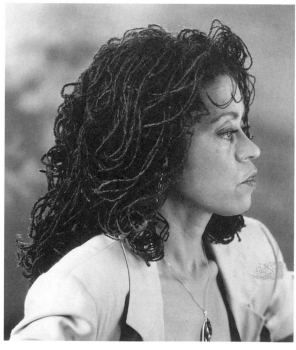

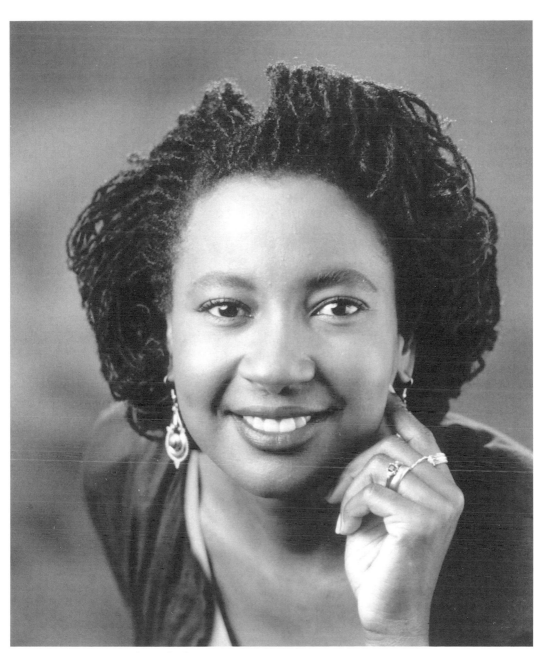

Photo courtesy Sisterlocks®

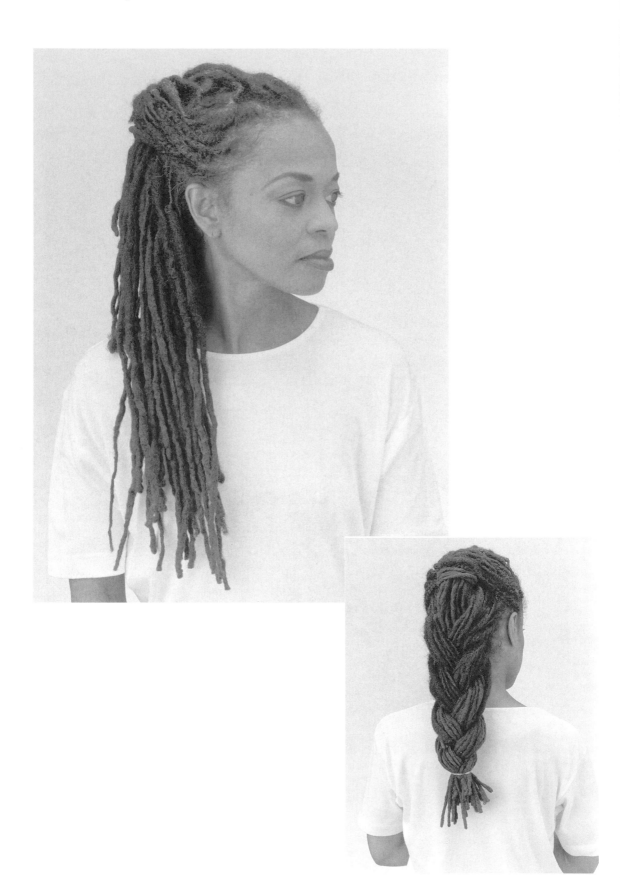

Details for Healthy Locks....

Too heavy locks -- Save your locks from breaking off.
Usually if your hair is naturally thick or more than eight years old, the locks will begin to feel heavy. A trim or lock cut will relieve the weight. Unless you have locked the hair for religious purposes, a cut is recommended. The hair will grow back; so look at it as a style change. Cut 2-6 inches off the locks to relieve the weight. Some clients have cut their waist length locks to a stylish shoulder length or even a chin length bob as an in-between style before completely cutting their locks off.

After you have invested years of growing beautiful long locks, the last thing you want is for them to begin breaking off at the scalp. If the lock becomes too thin (from age, wear and tear) at the base, you may need to double up and fortify the base hair so that you do not lose locks. One way to save a lock that is dangling on a thin piece of hair is to connect it to a more supported lock. You can double the weak-base lock to a thicker strong-base lock or if there is hair growing around the lock base, incorporate this into the thin lock base. To avoid this problem, establish good consistent grooming habits. Always palm roll the new grown hairs in one direction on the entire head. Do not handle the root hair more than every three weeks and be gentle when you massage during a shampoo.

Double Locks for Strength
1. When there is at least one inch of new growth between the scalp and lock, open the loose new growth hair into two parts.
2. Thread the end of the weak lock through the middle of the open new growth part of the strong base lock. (The joined locks may grow out forklike.)
3. If there is enough new growth hair around the thin base lock, twist or roll the hair into the thin lock to augment its base and make it thicker.
(For our male clients who have male pattern balding at the crown of the head, we have sewn a lock cut off from another area of the head to fill in the thinning spot.)

Smooth Edges
To give the hair line and front edges a neat appearance you may flatten the hair several different ways. Some clients who have high profile jobs need a neat, compact style. "Salon locks" are more for style than statement; so the finishing can give a distinct edge and professional look. Women, especially, may want a smooth, flat effect on the hairline. For a separated, individual braid effect; palm roll the hairline locks to tighten the loose hair growth and smooth the frizz. For a curly, wavy hairline; dampen the hair around the edges; use a natural water soluble gel or a light oil and rub a small amount onto the hair, then tie the hair firmly with a scarf or Hair Tucker™ band. Leave the hair tied flat for 20 minutes or overnight. When you remove the scarf or band, the hair is flattened with texture.

Lint Accumulation in the Locks

Lint can collect in your locks from blankets, sweaters and clothing. Choose wisely, the things you will lay your head upon and where your locks will have contact. Avoid wool blankets, mohair, or wool clothing that will rub into balls from friction of the locks rubbing against the material. If you have lint stuck in your locks, try to remove it immediately while the hair is dry. Gently stretch the locked hair and remove the lint. Examine your locks daily so that if you have lint or debris on the hair you can remove it right away. Once the hair has been shampooed, conditioned and oiled, the lint can work itself into the locks, making it more difficult to remove without tearing the lock apart.

If the lint is deeply imbedded in the lock, you can use a vegetable hair color rinse to color the hair and cover the lint. If you lighten the hair apply it to the lock ends. This gives a fashionable look as well as covers the lint build-up.

Breaking Midway

Avoid doing things that weaken your locks; such as, too vigorous scrubbing during the shampoo, frequent hair dying to lighten the locks and constant picking and bending of the locks. Dry hair that is not conditioned will deteriorate and weaken throughout the lock. Be mindful that the hair at the end of the lock is not connected to the scalp. Locks are formed by the hair matting and intermingling to form a cluster mass of hair. This hair, which would normally shed and be combed out, intertwines with the growing hair to make the lock. This formation is the reason the lock, especially if it is thin or of fine hair texture, becomes fragile and tears apart. So if the locks are disturbed and handled roughly, tearing and weakening in the middle of the lock is inevitable.

Mildew from Damp Locks

One of my male clients, who had three-year-old shoulder length locks, eventually cut off his locks because he felt they were ruining his clothing. He discovered that his damp locks were the cause of the mildew odor to his shirt collars. After shampooing or when the ends of your locks get wet in the shower, if they do not completely dry, the damp hair laying upon shirt collars or blouses will keep the fabric moist, causing mildew. If you have experienced this, it is best to shower with a shower cap to keep the lock ends from getting wet, and after a shampoo, allow enough time for the ends to dry completely or dry the ends using a blow dryer. Never sleep on damp hair, as it will cause a mildew on your pillows, and you increase the chance of developing a head cold. Sleeping on damp locks also will cause the locks to bend out of shape.

Product Build-Up

In your quest to grow healthy beautiful locks, someone told you to put bees wax, mud, gels, and whatever else on your hair. Now, all this gook has accumulated and embedded in your hair. As the hair locks, this build-up of gook will adhere to the matted hair. It will literally look like matted dirt, especially at the area where the hair has started to lock. If product build-up has been neglected for too long it will become impossible to remove. For hair that has not been coated too long with mud, gels, beeswax, etc., meticulously squeeze lathered shampoo throughout each lock. It will take numerous shampoos over a period of time, to remove the embedded dirt, and oil.

To remove product (residue) build-up:

1.) Rinse the hair with water as hot as you can tolerate.   **2.)** Shampoo with a de-greasing shampoo and continuously squeeze the lathered shampoo through the areas that have the concentrated build up.   **3.)** Rinse the hair with 1/4 cup apple cider vinegar or lemon juice mixed with 1 pint water. Final rinse with warm water.   **4.)** Roll the locks with a hand towel to dry and absorb any buildup. (Once you remove the build-up, select natural products that are light and water soluble. This will assure clean, light weight locks.)

Frequently asked questions

1. *Can I naturally lighten my locks?*
Other than the natural oxidation of hair from sunlight and other elements there are no natural products that are mild enough to remove the natural color from the hair. Some hair types will naturally lighten at the ends due to oxidation.

2. *Can permed hair lock?*
Locks are best formed with naturally curly, kinky hair. Relaxed hair is absent of curl, therefore it would be very difficult to form locks with twist or handrolls; however the with Sisterlock® method it is possible.

3. *Can I wear locks to the office?*
Many contemporary and sophisticated lock styles are appropriate for any work place. Women of diverse and ultra-professional positions are sporting their locks to work. Worn with the right attire, attitude and job knowledge, your locked hair should not become an issue in the workplace.

4. *Can I remove color tint from my salt-n-pepper locks?*
Once you apply color to white or graying hair, the hair is stained for the life of your locks. There is no process that can remove color from the hair bringing back the true color. You will have to cut off the colored locks and start from the beginning or grow out the locks with two tones covering the new growing hair with head wraps until you have enough new locks to cut off the colored ends.

5. *Why is my scalp constantly itchy?*
An itchy scalp is a sign that something is irritating the scalp. Change your hair care products and see if this makes a difference. Shampoo the hair more frequently, keeping the new growth hair moisturized and separated, so that the scalp may easily breath. Don't keep a damp scalp and check for head lice. Head lice will look like dandruff, but collects in clusters and does not brush off the hair. The eggs (nits) hold onto the hair with a glue like substance. Also, look closely for movement of the lice. If this is the problem, the best and only solution is to cut off all your hair. Generally, for loose hair, the head lice removal process is very tedious with hair strand combing required which is not possible with locked hair. Head lice is a more common problem with school age children or adults around a lot of children.

6. *Can I lock my naturally straight texture hair?*
All hair will tangle and matt which encourages the locking process. Straighter textures of hair can take upto 18 months to begin locking. With patience and the use of a stripping shampoo, it is possible to lock your naturally straight hair.

7. *How do I take the locks out?*
Hair locks are permanent; once you hair becomes rooted it is impossible to comb out the matted hair. If you are not sure you are ready to permanently lock the hair, wear wet, individual twist to create a similar style.

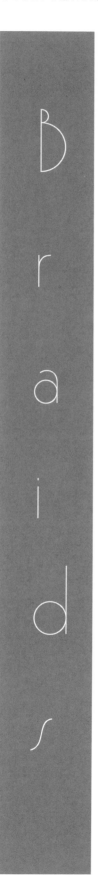

How to find a professional braider
Hair extensions
Braids, twist and handroll styles
Good grooming for braids

BRAIDS....BRAIDS....AMERICAN BRAIDS

Whether one braid or multiple braids, this ancient style transforms as black women's lifestyle and needs change. Braiding has its roots in Africa, but the African-American experience has influenced today's high fashion American style braids.

The American hair braider, unfamiliar with African techniques that can vary from region to region, has drawn upon what she learned in the African-American community with its rich cultural neighborhoods. A hodge-podge of creative energies can be found in American black neighborhoods, where girls practiced on baby doll's hair, each other and anything that had three pieces to braid.

Isolated from the larger culture in America, black neighborhoods are incubators for innovative hair fashion and some of the world's leading hair braiders. Some styles of braids in the black community often copied "white people's" hair styles. African-American hair braiders adapted their braid styles to swing, hang and give plenty of movement. They tried to make them soft to the touch and sometimes colored them with blond highlights, added red and gold extensions, or cut them in precision styles that would rival any European haircut. Coupled with intricate bead and thread embellishments, the style of braids in America are distinctly different from the styles done in Africa. African-American hair braiders created the American braid renaissance for both here and abroad.

As I look back at my early interest in hair braiding and the many gifted hair braiders I met, again, I feel the intense joys and pain of this growing and evolving industry. Braiding, in the late 1970's, was believed by mainstream America to be a trend that would not last long. How little they knew! Hair braiders knew different because we were working from ancestral foundations and could predict the demise of traditional cosmetology for black women.

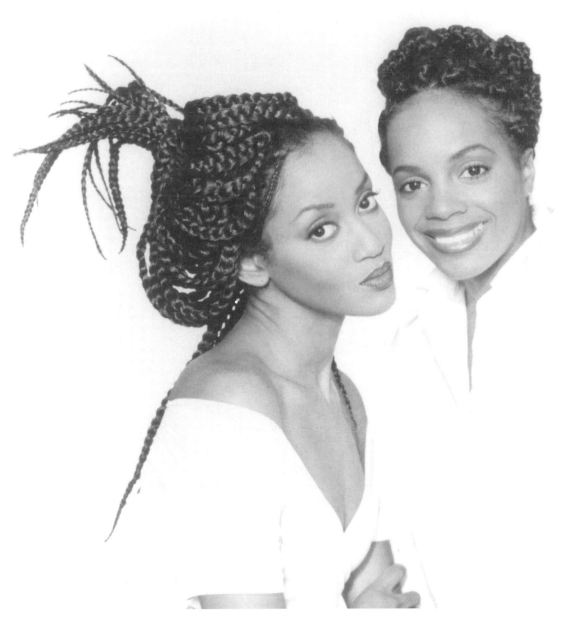

Soft Braids

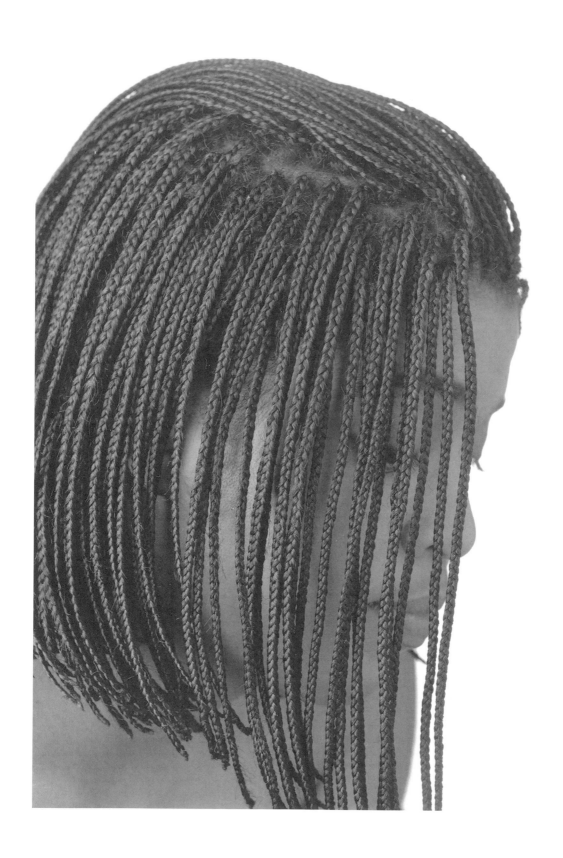

The cosmetology industry has become so obsessed with chemical hair care and European hair texture, that black women are experiencing burn out, burnt off hair, broken edges and a need to express their innate loveliness. Hair braiders are the alternative to "fix your hair like a white woman" beauticians. Also, black women discovered that braids encouraged hair growth. The braid style was the much needed prescription for giving processed hair a rest and growing healthy hair.

Hair braiders became healers who would doctor black women's damaged hair and bruised spirit. Black women would seek us out because they knew the hair braider would nurture their damaged hair back to health, even though some women would go and perm their hair time and time again. Braiders were sometimes frustrated, but continued to educate and teach black women to love their natural hair and African-inspired hair styles. In the process, the true American hair braider was born to set the standard for healthy hair care and alternative hair styling.

Part of the growing pains in the hair care industry was that braiders were looked down on by "Euro-educated" hair dressers and even the "uppity Negroes" who felt that braids were for the under-class. Many women changed their tune, once they started going bald and needed a braider to restore their hair. The American braider, looking for validation and recognition, found her own specialized place in the hair industry. Natural hair care via the black esthetic was her forte.

I can remember my first trip to West Africa in 1982, embracing Africa as the place to get some historical facts on the art of hair braiding. I thought I could easily find documentation, books and photo libraries full of information about the history of braids. I found, instead, that as in America, the history and nuances of the art of hair braiding are contained in a closed network of family braiders. Most of the African hair braiders I met were through personal introductions. They were pleasantly surprised and excited about the "American hair braider," and could not believe I learned how to braid in an American neighborhood in Providence, Rhode Island; not in Africa.

I realized, then, that my style of American braiding and hair care was quite advanced and unlike the African braiders. In studying the many styles of hair braiders throughout the United States, I found a distinct difference between the African hair braider's styles and methods and that of the American hair braider. For example, American hair braiders stand behind the head to invert braid, while the African hair braider stands in front of the head to produce the same braid. The American hair braider's beginning points for extension cornrows is flat, away from the hairline, to create a soft undetectable effect; while the African hair braiders' extension braid covers and in some cases creates a hairline, giving the effect of a sculpted cap.

American hair braiders generally braid to encourage hair growth; African braiders braid for style and culture. In some regions of Africa, the braids are often entirely too tight and cause bald receding hairlines. Hair care is not their main objective. (This is not to say that American braiders don't braid the hair too tight as well.) But the advent of natural hair was a direct result of the work of American hair braiders. However, despite the differences, we braiders were on equal footing and both had something to offer during my visits to Africa. We exchanged ideas, styles, methods, and techniques.

In America, African hair braiders have benefited from the popularity of African-American women who want their hair braided. They are able to earn a living, far greater than what they could make in Africa. Our African sisters have come to America and used their skills to capitalize on the growing hair braiding industry. The most successful African hair braiders are those who adapt to American standards and styles that African- American consumers desire.

How to find a professional hair braider

The biggest challenge to having your hair braided is finding a professional hair braider and hair braiding salon. Unfortunately, because there are few, if any, schools that teach the science of hair braiding, resources are limited. The traditional way of finding a qualified and experienced person in any practice is to start at the schools. But until a hair braider's license is available throughout the United States, finding hair braiders via schools is not an option. Word of mouth and seeing a beautiful style on someone else are two safe places to start.

If you see someone wearing a braid style you like, ask for the braider's telephone number. The most creative and skilled hair braider's work will speak for itself. Let the person who is wearing the braid style know that you are interested in finding a good braider to care for your hair. Some customers are selfish and do not share their braider's name, for some childish fear that you may get the same style. Don't let this discourage you; just keep your eyes open for beautifully braided hair styles and continue to ask until you get the name of the best hair braider in your area.

In your quest for finding a good hair braider, don't get so desperate that you go to a girlfriend's cousin's sister's house "to get your hair did" for twenty dollars. Too often, cheap, braided hair styles look like you were used as a practice head. They have big knots, frizzy braids, no style and just plain tacky looking. Expect to invest in your hair care.

The other problem you may encounter is the home braiders house or even some shoddy braid salons that may be in the worst of conditions and circumstances. It all depends on your tolerance level. I have had clients tell me about their experience with some of the most talented braiders who live in unsafe neighborhoods, their houses may not be in the most sanitary condition, babies may be running around the house and who knows what else. You make the choice of going through this to have your hair braided. Women have complained that some braiding salons are expensive, but the difference may be in service, atmosphere and hygiene.

In major cities across the United States, braid salons are opening at a fast rate. All braiding salons, however, are not created equal. Beware of the braid salons that have become sweat shops that offer bargain prices from unskilled workers. The old saying, "you get what you pay for," holds true for cheap braid styles done by untrained braiders who know little about sanitation or hair and scalp care. Some braiders can braid nicely but know little about how to take care of your hair. You will have to be the judge from your first impression and overall comfort with a new salon and braider.

Some things you may look for are whether the salon is clean, organized, and stocked with the products and supplies for braiding your hair. Ask for a consultation, so that you may look at photos of their work and get answers to questions that concern your hair needs. If the salon has novice or apprentice hair braiders, ask if they will be supervised by an experienced hair braider. This may help you avoid a bad braid experience.

During the consultation, give any details about past braid experiences, whether you will be swimming, exercising and need style versatility or low maintenance. Explain your style likes and dislikes; (for example, you may not like hair off your face). The more a stylist knows about you the easier it is to create a style to suit your needs.

Questions to ask a braider during a pre-braid consultation.

1. May I see photos of styles that you have done here? (Some braider photo albums will include pictures from magazines, books and work not done at the salon.)
2. Based on my texture and hair condition, is my hair strong enough to braid?
3. Can you tell me the pros and cons of the braid styles I like.
4. How much will the style cost and how long will it take to braid?
5. How long will the style last before I should have it rebraided?
6. What types of extensions will be used; human hair or synthetic fiber and is this included in the total price?
7. Do you shampoo and condition my hair before braiding?
8. How should I take care of my braided style?
9. How should I remove the braids before re-braiding?
10. How much will it cost to have it re-braided?

Choosing the Right Hair Extensions

Hair extensions have their place in styling and grooming. The naturalist may use them occasionally to achieve a certain style, give the natural hair a rest, for longevity or to add length to a braid style. If you have long, healthy hair, however, I recommend using extensions sparingly. Hair extensions can become just as addictive as chemical processing. Their use should be limited so that the hair can be managed and maintained naturally.

In the case where you may need to use extensions for in-between stages of growing out short, damaged or processed hair; to cover balding, thin areas, hair extensions are useful. Not only will they cover problem hair, but will protect your hair as it is growing.

Many American women are, for the first time, experimenting with hair extensions. Although relatively new in modern hair styling, extensions have been around for centuries. Egyptian women, like Cleopatra, are remembered for their elaborately braided wigs and military headdress made out of natural and artificial materials. The women of antiquity used hair extensions to protect their shaved heads from the hot sun. And even today, throughout Africa, you will still find women who wear hair extensions for traditional and ceremonial styles.

As with any hair care regimen, wearing hair extensions has its good and bad points. If you are wearing hair attachments for the first time or want to know how your hair additions can look as natural as possible, here are some tips that will help you make the right choice.

1. Always have hair extensions applied by a skilled, expert hair braider.

2. Select the right color, length and extension type, in consult with your braider, so that your new extension hair does not look artificial and obviously longer.

3. When the braids get frizzy and ratty looking, it is time to take out and re-do your hair extension style.

4. If hair extensions are applied correctly they will not pull the hair or hurt.

5. *The two types of hair extensions used for styling are weft and bulk.*
   a) **Weft** hair extension is loose hair sewn and bound together at one end, creating a band. The weft type extension is used for weaving and hair pieces.

   b) **Bulk** hair extension is a bundle of loose hair that is not permanently bound together. This type of extension is used to braid small pieces onto the hair.

6. There are many shades and colors of hair extensions. The most commonly used ones are universal for wigs and extensions, both human hair and synthetic fiber.

The advantage with human hair is that the hair can be colored any shade. However, the lighter the color the more it will cost due to processing or limited raw hair. On the other hand, synthetic fiber cannot be colored. It comes in a fair range of colors that are plentiful and inexpensive and all colors, including blondes, cost the same.

Hair Extension Colors.

Below are some standard colors used in the hair industry.
Hair extension colors are referred to by number
The lower the number the darker the color.

Number	Color	Number	Color
1	black	27-30	light auburn & blonde
1B	off black	33	burgundy red
2	dark brown	280	15% gray
3	medium brown	34	brown mixed gray
4	auburn brown	51	50% gray
6-8	ash light brown	16-22	pale blonde

Extension textures

Human hair and synthetic fiber extensions come in a broad selection of textures. This gives you the choice to match your hair texture closely or to choose a hair texture that is totally different from your own. The great advantage of using textured hair extensions is that you can sample different hair textures without permanently and chemically altering your natural hair.

The most common hair textures are wet and wavy, curly, spiral curl, zig zag, krimpy, body wave and straight. The Afro texture hair extension is workable as a hair piece, or braided into small lace braids, however as a weave it requires special maintenance. It has been impossible to duplicate Afro hair that has the same flexibility and characteristics of real hair. The problems have been tangling, drying, coarseness and lacking good elasticity so that the hair can be combed, stretched or straightened to revert to the Afro curl. It does not resemble natural hair which is soft, spongy, and elastic.

Human hair extensions are purchased from live persons who grow their hair to sell it and not cut from dead people. Human hair has become a commodity in a time when appearance is so important. The quality, texture and color of the human hair extension may vary, depending on the original condition of the person's hair and how the hair is gathered. For instance, some hair is gathered from combings while better quality hair is cut directly from the head and maintained in that order. The best human hair is hair that is in the same direction it grows from the head. The hair cut closest to the root hair is the cuticle end and the open end is the hair end.

Where the hair comes from and how it is processed makes a difference in the finished quality of human hair extensions. The raw human hair is generally obtained from parts of Europe, the Orient, Indonesia and India. Quality can range from the finest, which has good luster, elasticity, feels soft, curls easily and handles well. Poor quality hair is dry, brittle, stiff, dull in color and does not hold a curl or is too rough to style.

The refining process, which involves sanitizing, coloring and texturing, can give second-quality hair good characteristics. This all depends on the products used for refining the hair and the skill of the person processing it. With modern processing, we can expect the quality of imported

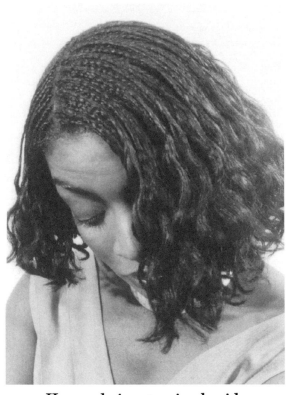

Human hair extension braids

processed hair to improve, giving you a quality human hair extension at a fair price. Although more costly, the best quality human hair is processed in America.

The more knowledgeable you become about judging the qualities of human hair, the better able you will be to prevent purchasing dry, matting and stiff human hair. Usually these characteristics surface after the first shampoo. Some things to consider about human hair extensions are whether the hair feels soft, can be easily combed through with your fingers, and does not drip the dye color nor become stiff after it gets wet. These things can be tested before braiding or weaving the hair into your own. The last thing you want to do is sit for hours having your hair done with hair that will tangle after the first shampoo. Although the human hair extension is soft, natural and easier to manage, one disadvantage is that it easily loosens, because of its soft texture.

Tips to keep human hair extension braids from frizzing and loosening.
1. Shampoo no more than once a week.
2. When showering do not wet through to the scalp everyday. Cover your crown area with a shower cap. There is no harm done if the ends get wet daily.
3. Human hair extensions are not recommended for short or blunt cut hair.
4. Do not apply to freshly relaxed hair.
5. Not recommended for frequent swimming.
6. Do not put grease, gels or heavy oil on human hair extensions.

As with all hair extensions there are risks involved. Whether human or synthetic, the hair is treated by a chemical process. Unfortunately, there are no chemical ingredients listed on the packs of hair extensions you may use. So you risk not knowing what your skin and scalp may come in contact with. I have found, through tests, that some human hair extensions are dyed with products that contain the chemical Phenylenediamine. This chemical is known to cause eczema, skin rash, bronchial asthma and death. Poisoning can occur through scalp absorption. Even though there is not enough information to prove or disprove that this chemical can cause cancer in humans, the American Cancer Society cautions against the use of substances that are in question and have not been thoroughly tested.

(If you experience unexplained scalp irritation, extreme itching, circulatory problems or asthma, discontinue use of the extensions immediately.)

Animal hair extensions are sometimes mixed in with human hair extension. Would you be surprised to learn you may be wearing animal hair or a combination of human and animal hair extensions? Unscrupulous hair dealers and lax controls allow for the sale of animal (yak) hair as 100 percent human hair. Only a trained eye and hand can distinguish the real differences. These dealers depend on you having no idea that animal hair can be disguised as human hair.

Animal hair comes from the angora goat, ox (yak), horses and sheep. Because animal hair can be difficult to work with, it is usually mixed with low quality human hair. The angora hair is usually soft and fine, while the horse and sheep hair is coarse and very straight. This hair is plentiful and cheap. It is recognized by its coarse dry texture and matting and stiffening after a shampoo. So the next time you buy human hair and it is very inexpensive, mats, tangles and looks stiff, it is likely that animal hair has been mixed in.

Synthetic fiber has come a long way. Although it does not have the easy style versatility of human hair, if it is done in the salon by a skilled hair braider, it can resemble human hair. Synthetic fiber is a plastic resin manufactured to resemble the textures, colors, sheen and feel of real hair. It is non-absorbent and lacks porosity so it may cause itching because the scalp cannot breathe through the synthetic fiber; however, if you are not sensitive to this, it is durable and holds the braid style well. Synthetic hair is also processed with chemicals, so sensitivity and irritation may result for some people.

Braid styles which incorporate bob braids, burnt ends, corkscrew twists and permanent hot dipped curls, only synthetic fiber can be used. It is the molded plastic that permanently holds the shape. Beware that some synthetic fibers are flammable. Plentiful, inexpensive and popular for hair braiding, this fiber can be very damaging to the hair if used incorrectly.

Unskilled braiders often use to much extension, causing excessive weight on the natural hair, resulting in breakage. I have seen braiders use as many as twelve packs of hair for a braid style. This is unnecessary and extremely uncomfortable. To keep open synthetic ends from matting and looking "wiggy," brush daily. Do not use hot-temperature styling tools because it will burn and melt, causing the synthetic extension to feel hard. Synthetic extensions shampoo well; however, because they are not absorbent, it may take longer for the thicker braid styles to dry. Many transitional styles are done with synthetic fiber and the ultimate objective of its use is style durability.

Lin fiber is a hair extension attachment made from wool, cotton and synthetic material. It feels cottony and looks soft and puffy like African-American hair. This fiber is mostly used for rhasta twist, corkscrew styles and occasionally braids.

As the hair grows healthy, the true naturalist will eventually get rid of the hair extensions, forget about hair attachments and wear her own beautiful natural hair, which is what I wholeheartedly encourage.

Braids, Flat Twist and HandRoll Styles

This next section will show different styles that should be done by a skilled braider. The twist and hand roll styles are for natural hair. The cornrow and individual braid styles can be done on natural or chemically treated hair. Some styles take only an hour while more intricate styles, like small individual braids, can take up to eight hours. The distinct difference is that the styles that take the longest will last longer. Enjoy and explore the many style options on the following pages. These are just a few styles available for your hair.

Single braids

Braids, singles, plaits individuals, box, bob and micro braids are all individually sectioned braids. They are similar in technique but different in style, such as size, stitch and finishing. Because the hair is in small sections, this style of braids can be gathered, moved and easily manipulated.

Box braids are single braids parted in triangle, square or some other geometric shape. It gets its name from the way the section is parted.

Bob braids are single braids in a very stiff, tight stitch, burnt on the ends, giving the braids a permanent curve. Because of the tight stitch; this style braid is the most durable and is recommended for swimming and frequent shampoos.

Micro braids are the most misinterpreted braid style. Micro means small, not invisible. It is the finest, smallest braid one can make (too small a braid will break the hair). Also, the (micro) short braid can be braided one inch down and the rest of the hair extension is left loose.

Invisible braids also known as lace braids -- are like the individual braid method except that the loose hair extension covers the braid.

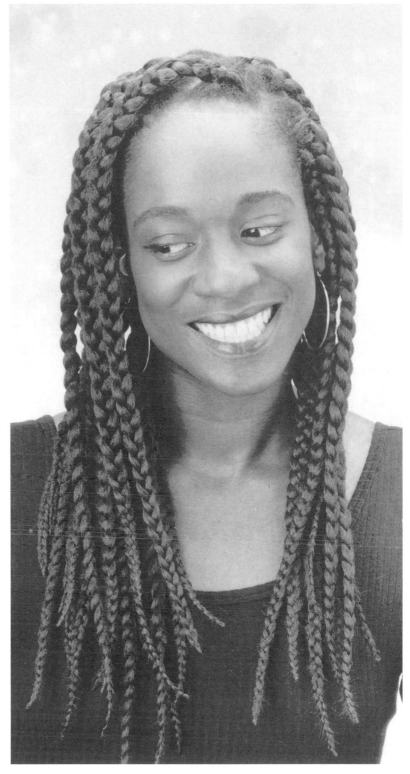

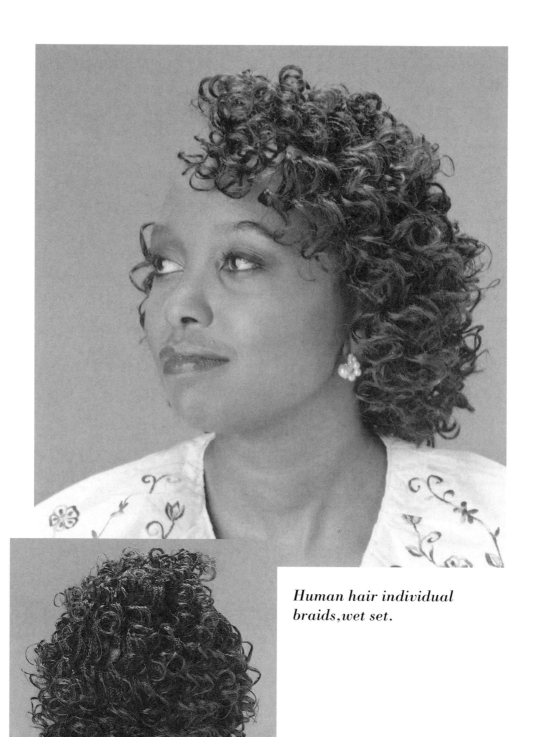

Human hair individual braids, wet set.

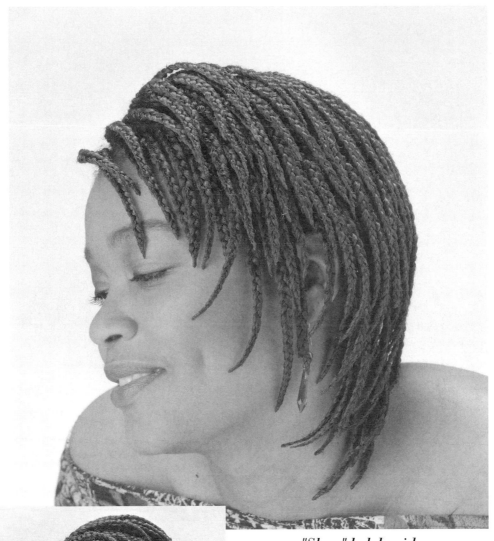

"Shag" bob braids

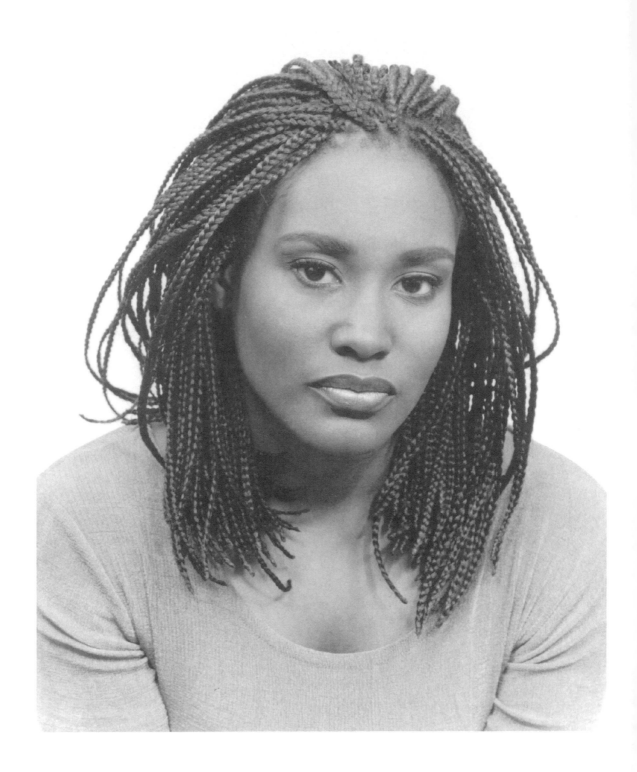

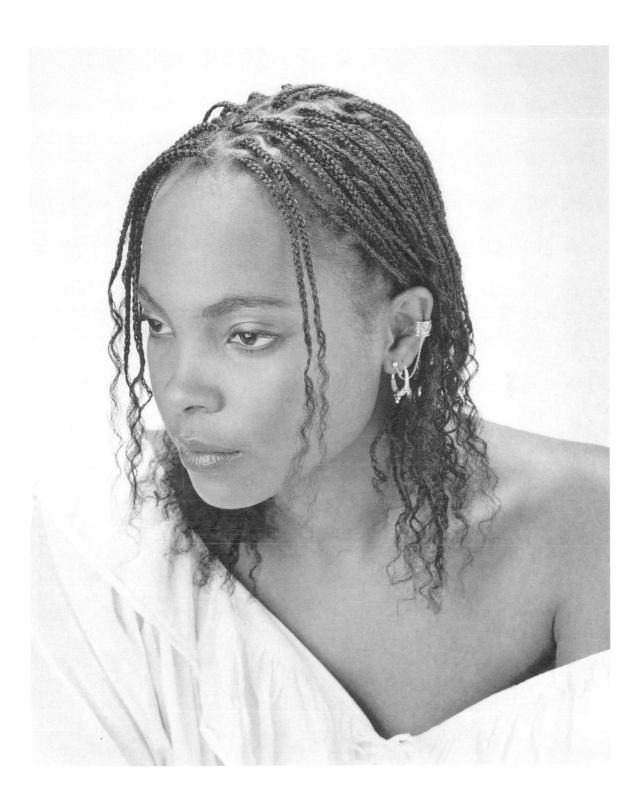

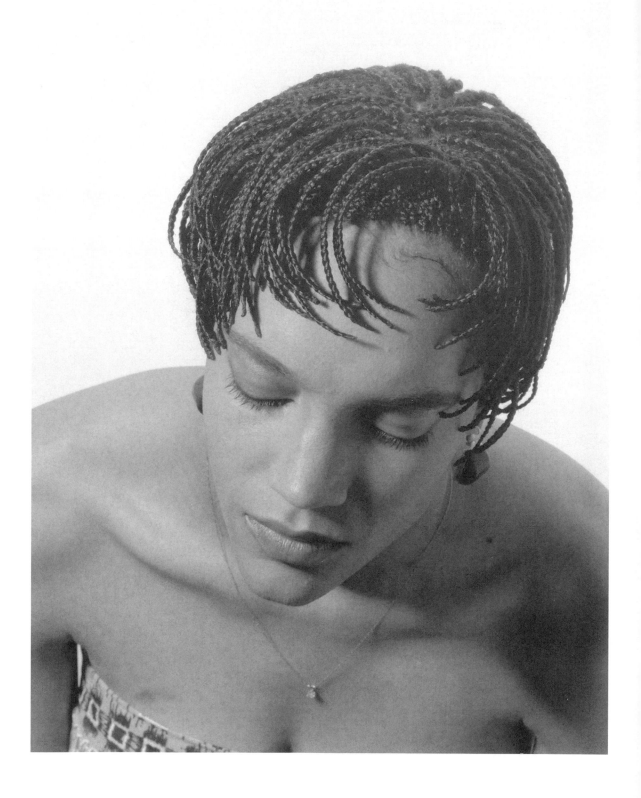

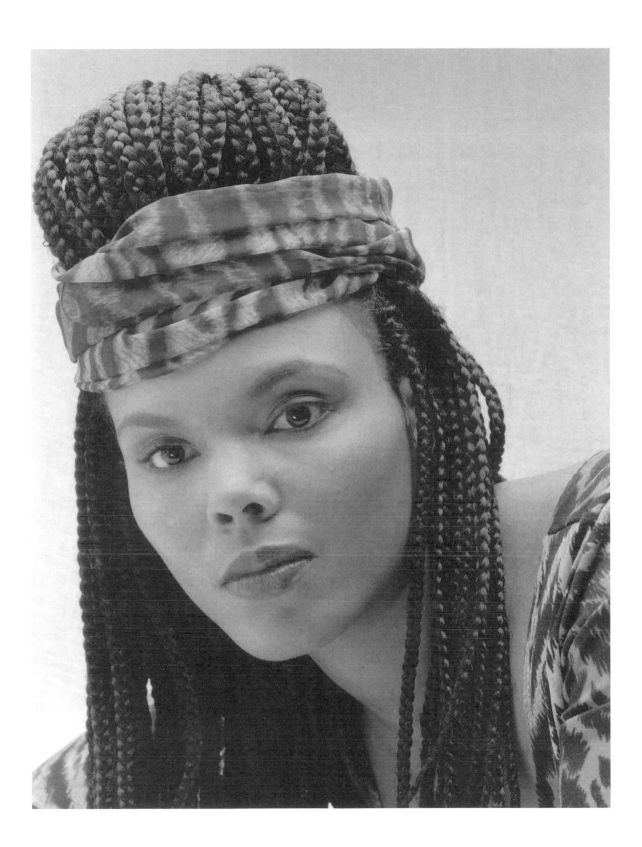

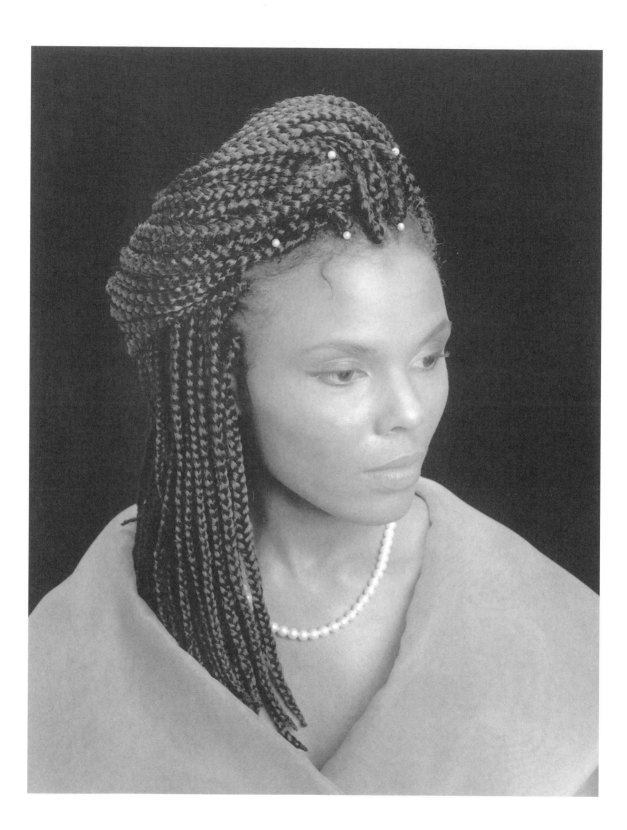

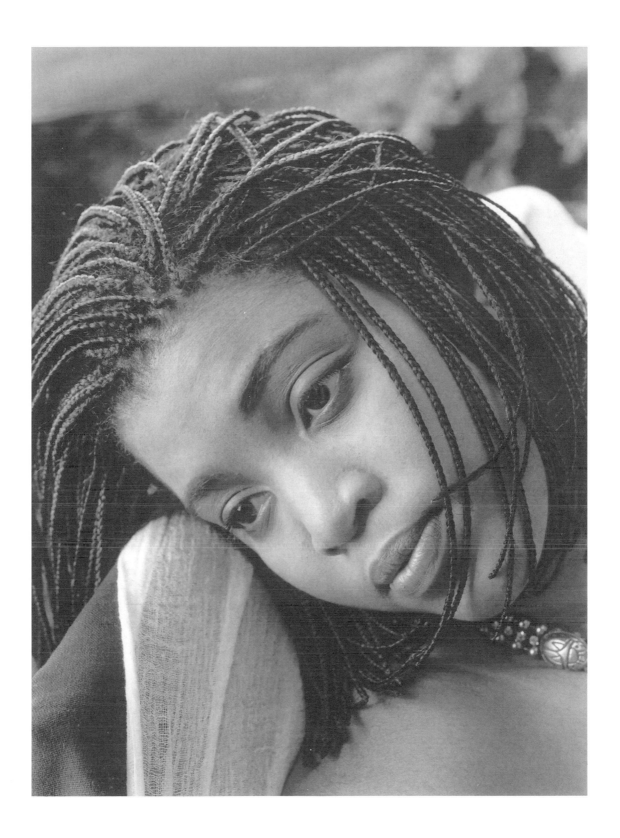

Cornrows

The cornrow is believed to get its name from the braids resemblance to planted rows of corn. In some American cities, the cornrow is also called a cornbraid, perhaps getting its name from the close appearance of neat rows of corn on the cob. The term will differ from region to region in America. Whether it is called cornrow or cornbraid, the terms are purely African-American.

There are several styles of cornrow braids -- the flat invert, outward, knitrows, thickrow and goddess. The method is the same for achieving these styles, except some cornrows are done overhand while others are underhand. Some are small, thick and very large. In general, the cornrow is a stationary braid that lays flat against the scalp. It can be done where the scalp is exposed between each braid or braided close together so you do not see any, parts between each row. Knitrows are cornrows that are intricately braided close together with no visible part, completely covering the scalp. At close view, it appears like a knitted texture.

The stationary cornrow style is great if you want a style that does not move out of position like the individual braids. This style is best done by a braid stylist. It is difficult to do on yourself, since the parting is fundamental to the styles accuracy and beauty. As shown on the following pages, cornrows can be worn for conservative, practical and the most professional lifestyles.

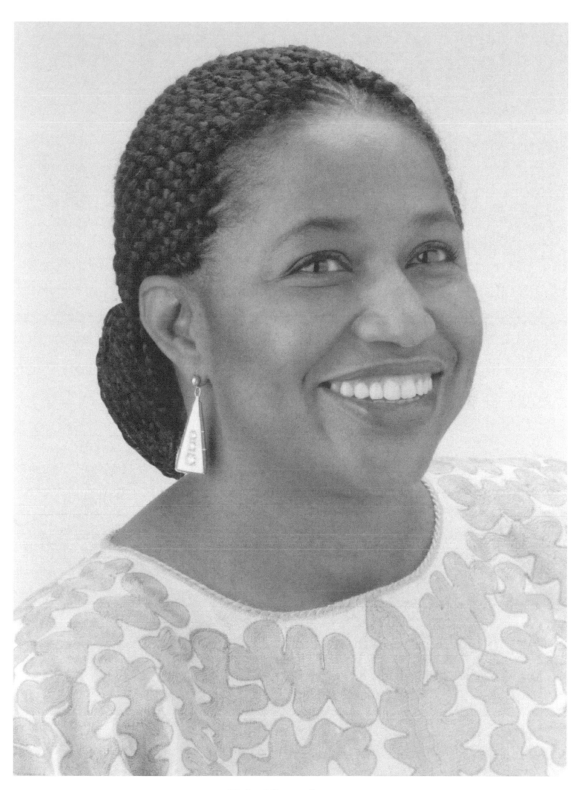

United States Senator
Carol Moseley-Braun

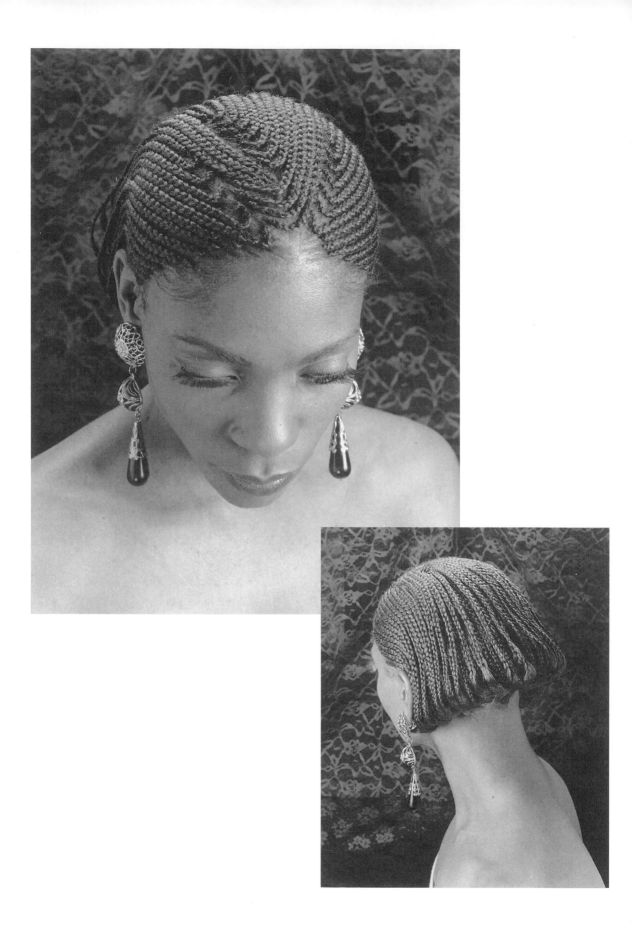

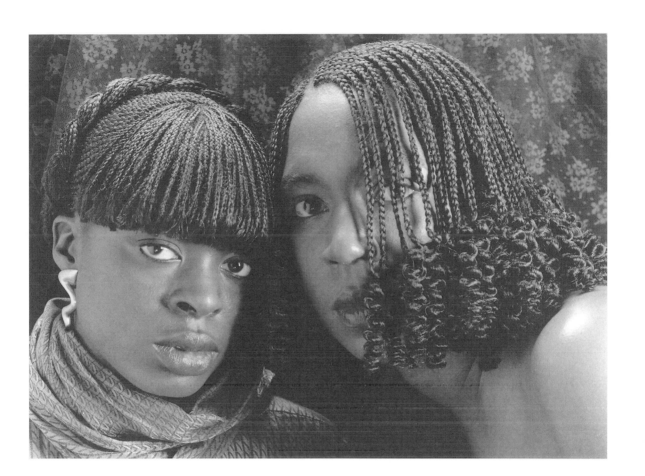

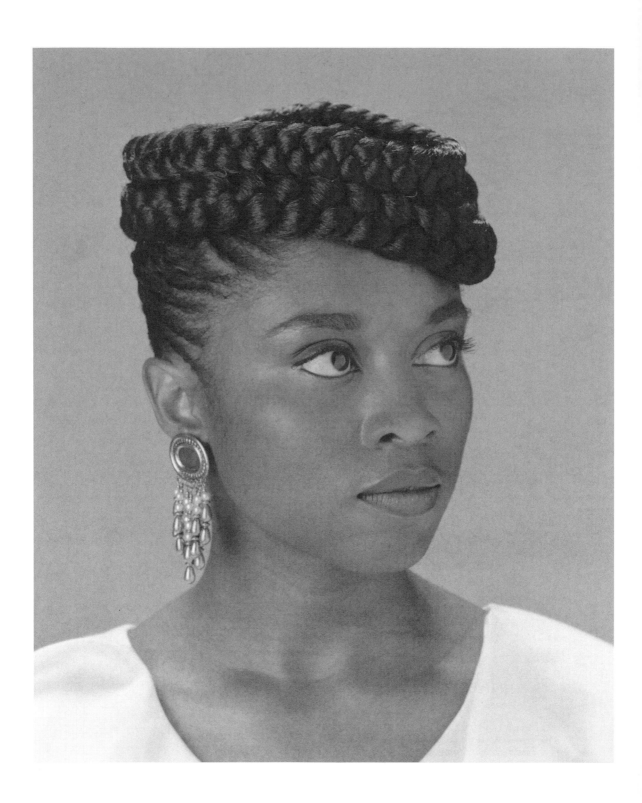

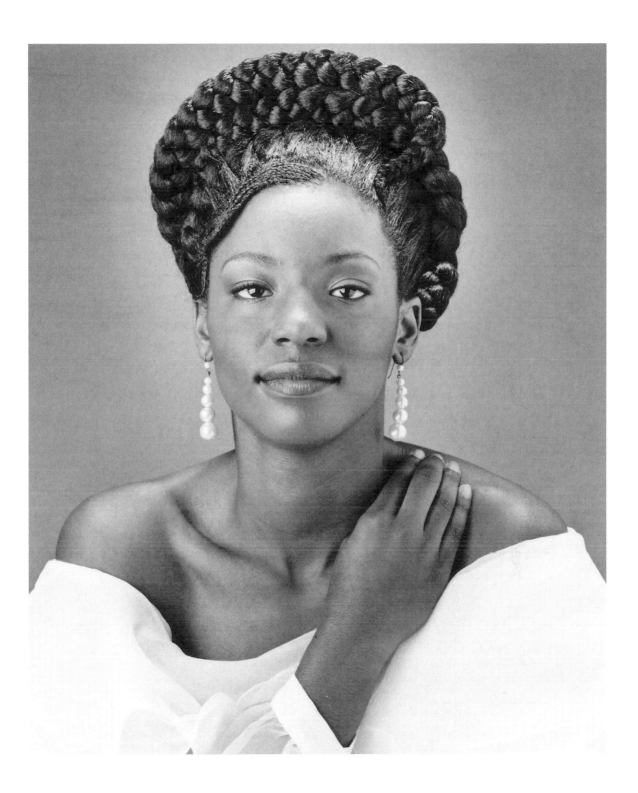

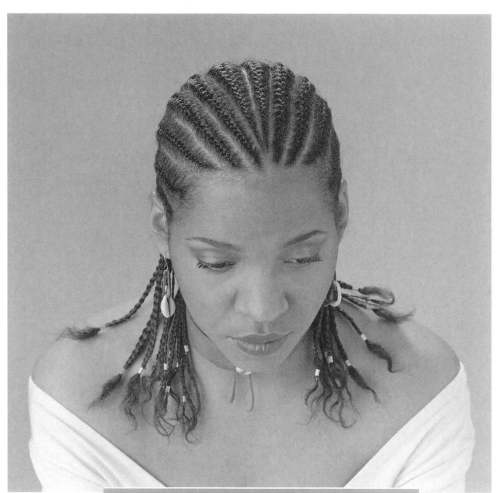

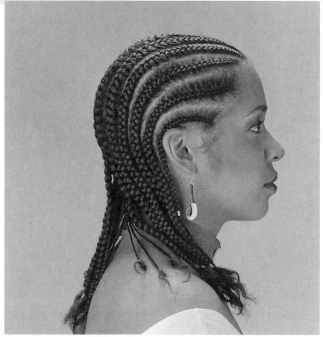

"Flat braid" cornrows

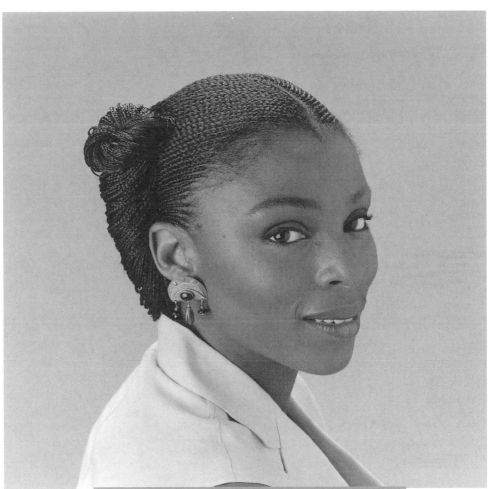

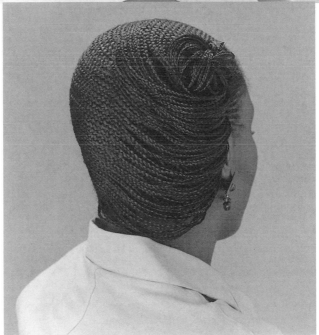

"Knitrows"

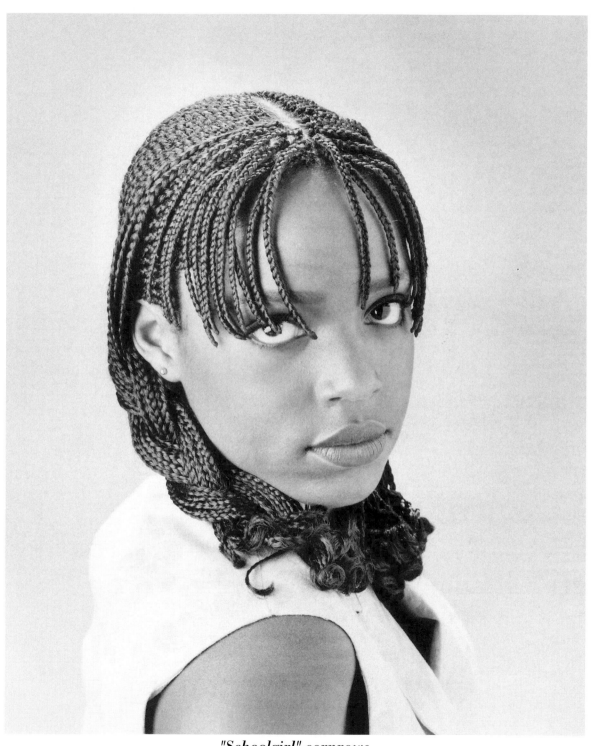

"Schoolgirl" cornrows

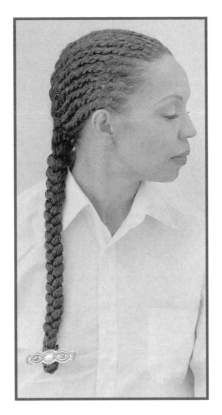

Flat twist

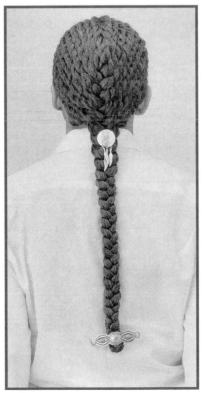

The flat twist style is similar to the corn-row, except the twist is done using two sections of hair. This quick style is a perfect option for longer natural hair. Most contemporary styles done on straight texture hair can be simulated with the flat twist technique. The shape and form of contemporary styles can be duplicated and the twist adds dimension with its raised rows of soft interlaced hair.

The twist is wonderful if you have been wearing braids with extensions and are ready to wear your own hair. The true benefit of the flat twist is that it is stationary and requires little maintenance other than tying the hair at bedtime. The flat twist is quick and painless to create, usually taking two hours or less to complete; including a shampoo. The style will stay neat one to two weeks or from shampoo to shampoo. (Shampooing is recommend weekly or bi-weekly.) The variety of twist styles are countless, depending on each person's hair and preferences.

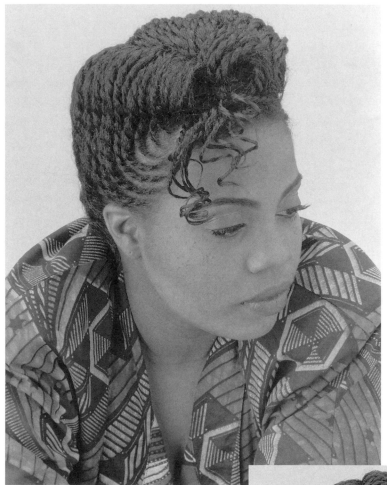

"Soft rolls"

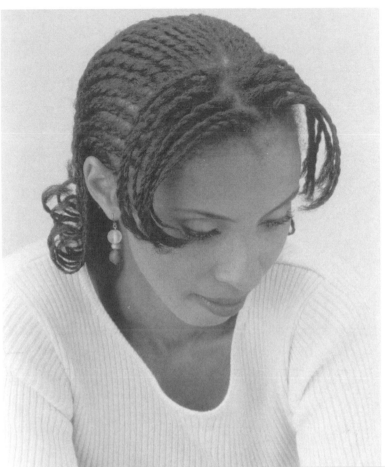

Flat twist "flip"

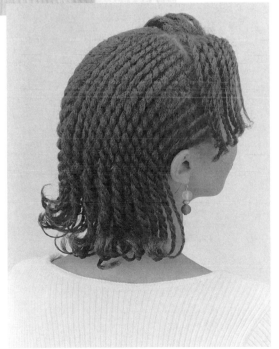

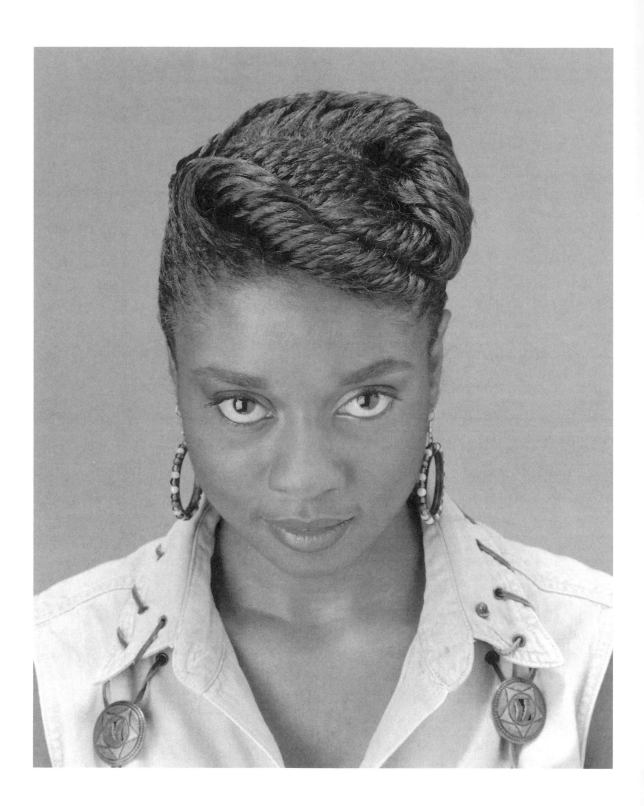

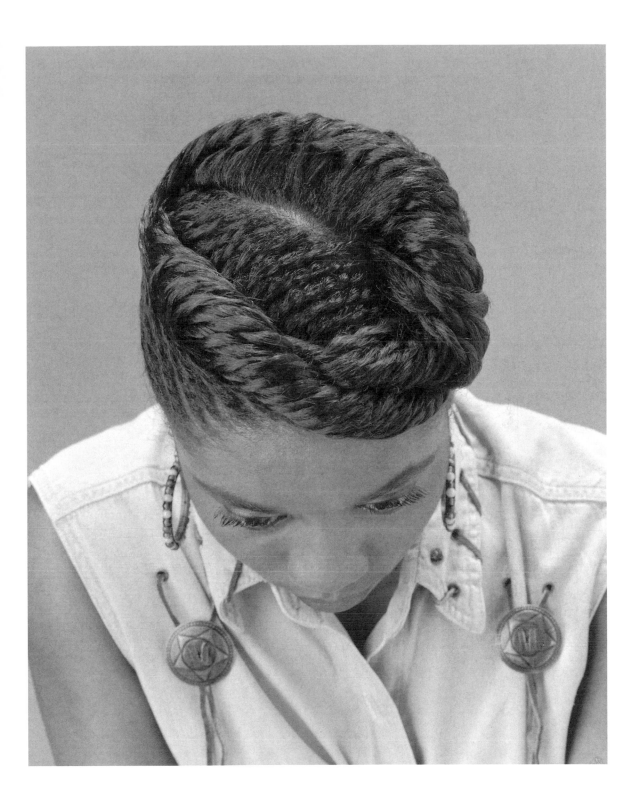

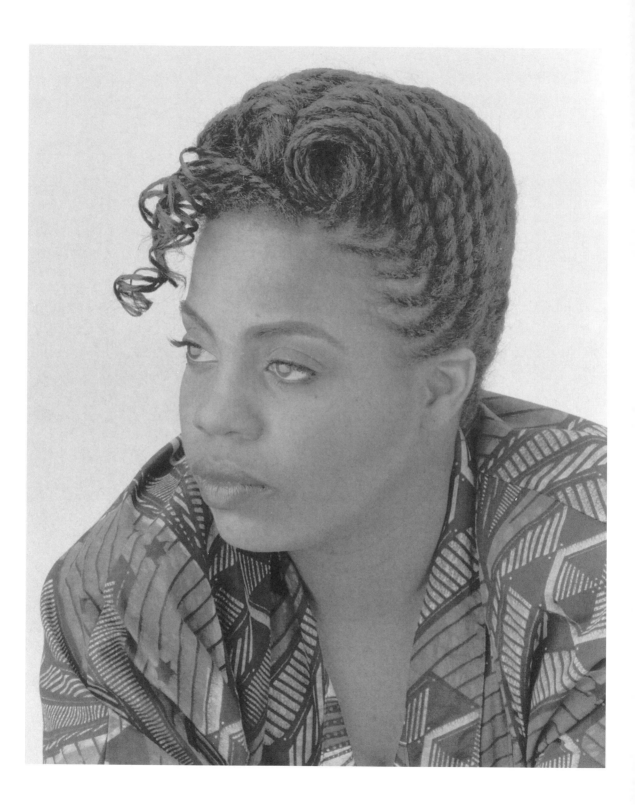

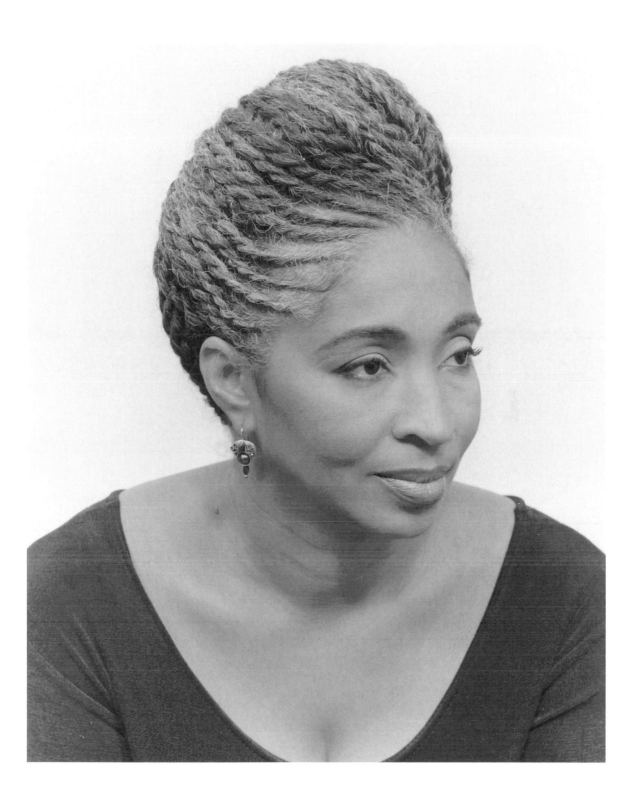

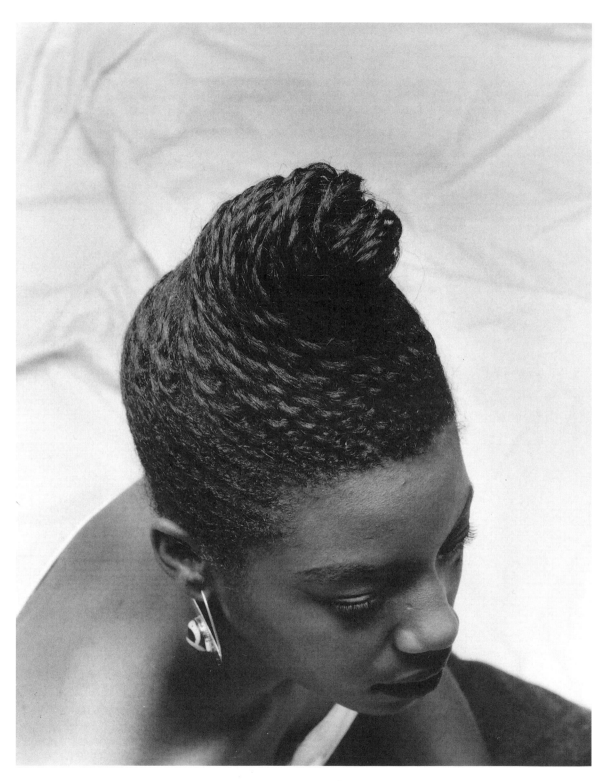

Flat twist "high roll"

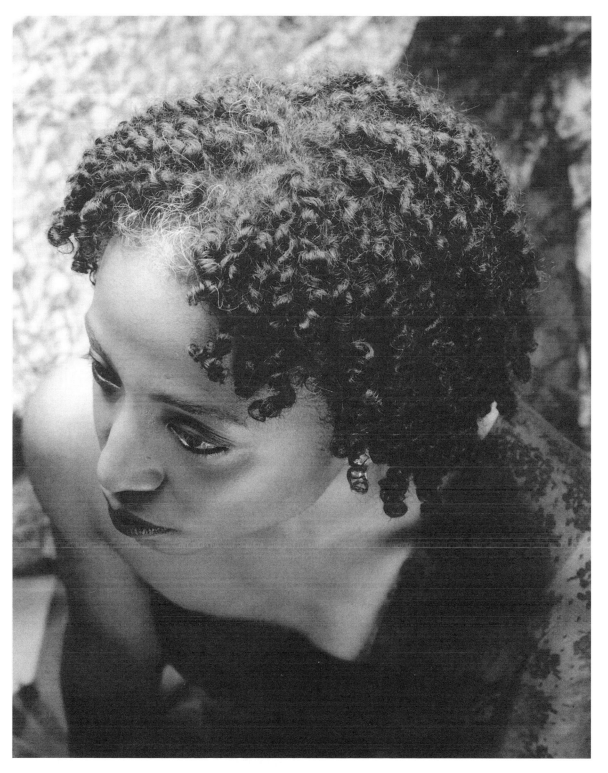

Individual Twist

Handrolls

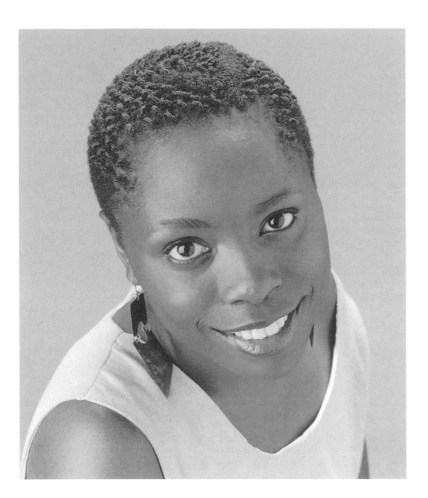

Imagine creating a perfect, durable curl without using rollers, curling irons, hair pins, etc. Handrolls are made using the natural curly coil in your hair. Rolls can add definition and drama to the short bush as it is growing longer and will give texture to the most curly, kinky hair. The natural curl in the hair is what holds the handroll in place.

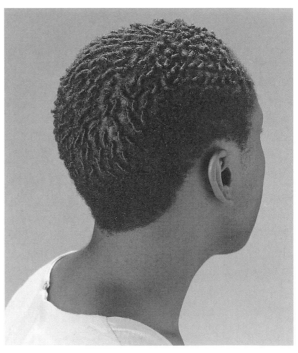

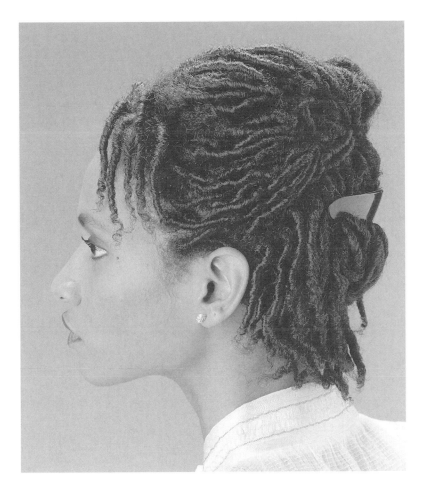

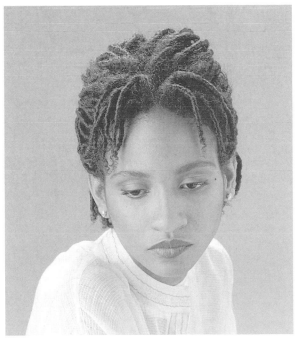

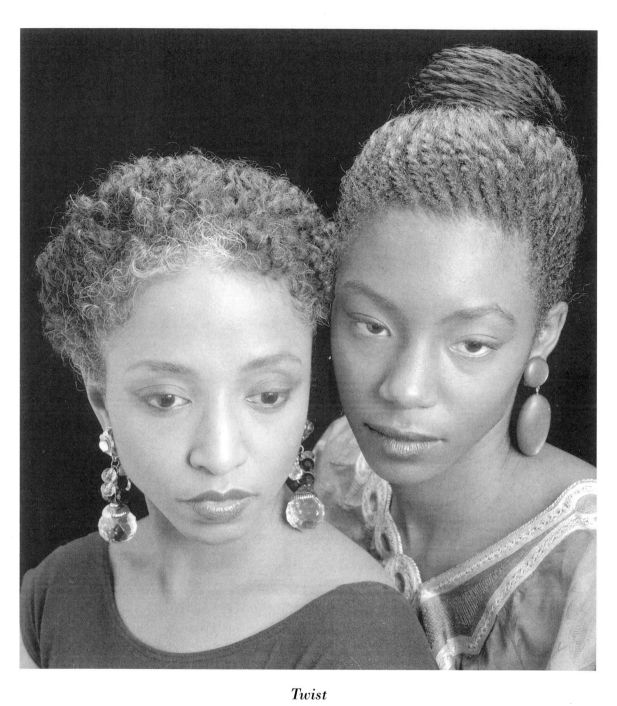

Twist

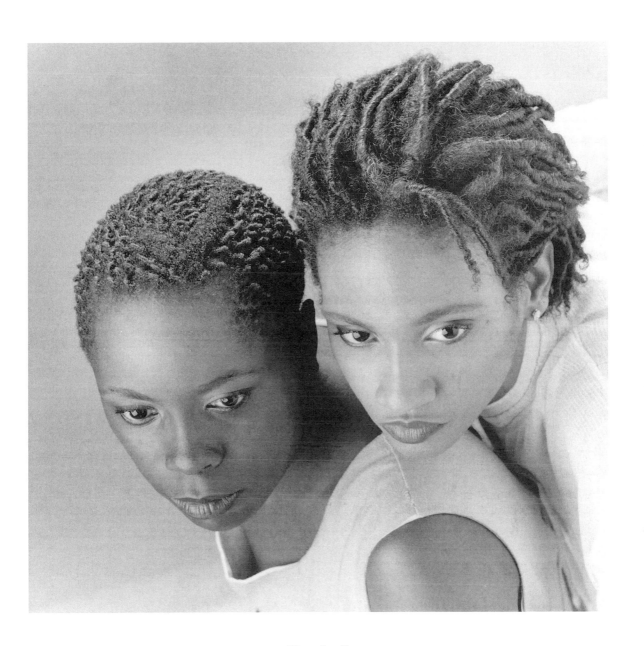

Handrolls

Good Grooming

Good grooming habits are essential to the most beautifully kept braid styles and it is your responsibility to keep your braid style in the best possible condition. If you are braiding your hair because you want a hair style that you don't need to care for, you are mistaken. Braids require grooming, styling and care like any other hair style. When they look bad or unkempt, unfortunately, people judge all braids based on the tacky, raggedy looking ones; even though they never comment on the chewed-up, broken off permed hair. So it is especially important for you to keep your scalp clean, your braids neat and the overall style neat and fresh looking.

When it is close to the time to have your hair re-braided, and your hair line appears to be growing out or the style is not as neat as it should be, use fashionable head wraps to camouflage or complement your braid style until your next braid appointment.

Night care

The first thing you will need to do after having your hair braided is protect it at bedtime. Tie a silk or cotton scarf over the cornrows to keep them neat and flat. For full volume braid styles, a slumber cap will do. To preserve the curled ends, use a scarf large enough to cover them. If the scarf does not stay on at bedtime, sleep on a satin pillow or follow the instructions "To stop hair frizz" (below) in the morning.

To stop hair frizz

All hair textures may frizz or fray out of the braid. This natural occurrence is sometimes beyond the control of the most skilled braider. Certain styles can be created with this in mind in order to keep frizzing at a minimum. While it is true that chemical relaxers will reduce chances of hair frizzing, it is in no way recommended or suggested that you do this to your hair. The risk of you losing your precious strands of hair from chemical relaxers is not worth no-frizz hair. Natural hair may frizz more often with cornrows and human hair extensions. Since water and humidity encourage the natural hair to curl and frizz, you may notice the most hair frizz after a shampoo. To flatten and reduce hair frizz:

1. **Dampen a soft bristle brush; gently brush the braids in the direction they are braided. (Angle the brush on a slant to prevent snagging the hair.)**

2. **Rub a small amount of recommended hair gel in the hands (no more than twice a week),then rub over the surface of the braids.**

3. **Tie the braids flat with a cotton scarf for 15 minutes; once you remove the scarf the frizz should be flat.**

How long should you wear your braid style?

Most cornrow and extension braids styles will remain neatly braided from four to eight weeks. Very small individual braids may last up to 12 weeks. Of course, this will depend on your particular style, hair texture, overall condition, and growth rate; provided you groom and care for your hair regularly. And if you do regular exercise and swim, your braided hair style may not stay neatly braided the full time. These circumstances may require having your hair re-braided more often than usual. Be sure to plan for this and not leave your hair braided if it does not appear neat and well groomed.

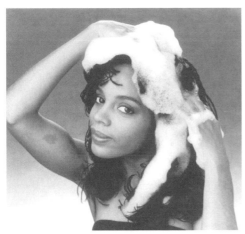

Lather a small amount of shampoo out to your finger tips and massage the scalp gently.

How to shampoo your braids

Your braid hair style should be shampooed at least once a week or bi-weekly.

1. Wet your braided hair under a gentle shower.
2. Lather a small amount of shampoo out to your fingertips and massage the scalp gently, between the braids, in the direction the hair is braided. (shampoo twice)
3. Thoroughly rinse out all of the shampoo (Conditioning is optional.)
4. Pat dry with a towel to remove as much excess water as possible.
5. If necessary, to flatten hair frizz, brush in the direction that the hair is braided.
6. Tie the hair with a large scarf so the hair will dry flat and look neat.

The ends of the braids can be set on rollers or after the hair has dried you may use an electric curling iron to re-curl human hair extensions. *Note*: Synthetic hair is curled different than human hair extensions. Ask your braider how to maintain the ends of your synthetic braids.

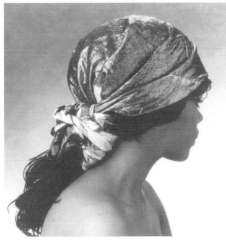

Tie the hair with a large scarf so the hair will dry flat.

Give your braids sheen

Unless your scalp is extremely dry, it is not necessary to oil between each braid. Do not use artificial oil sprays, activator, gels greases or lotions on your cornrows or on the scalp; this will cause a build-up on your hair. The other reason for avoiding these oils is that they can cause the hair to feel gummy and smell rancid and stale. Spray oils also have either alcohol or other chemicals in the product to thin the oil enough to spray. If you shampoo weekly, oil your braided hair no more than twice a week. With infrequent shampooing, oil less often. Remember that oil does not give moisture (it can maintain moisture), so if the hair and scalp are dry, regular shampooing will add moisture.

1. **Rub a dime size amount of light liquid natural oil in your hands.**
2. **Rub your oily hands onto the surface of your braids, in the same direction that the hair is braided.** *Note:* **Do not apply hair oil to loose human hair extensions; this will cause the hair to become flat and stringy. Oil the hairline, since this area may dry from daily washing of your face.**

Care for lace or interlock braids

Lace and interlock braid styles show a minimal amount of braids and give the illusion of loose hair. A soft textured extension (synthetic or human hair) is braided onto the natural hair. Because of the loose hair extension, these styles require special care during shampooing. To prevent tangling and dulling, select products that are mild and suited for hair extensions. During the first two weeks, hair will shed; so always comb out the hair before a shampoo. If possible, allow up to two weeks before the first shampoo or thorough wetting of the scalp.

1. **With fingertips, gently massage the lathered shampoo into the scalp working it through the extension hair lengthwise. (Never scrub the ends of the hair together as this will surely cause tangling.)**
2. **Rinse thoroughly and apply a rinse-out conditioner.**
3. **Towel blot excess water, allow the extension hair to air dry and place into your desired hair style.**

If you are wearing wavy hair extensions, to maintain the wave, comb daily with a large tooth comb then moisten the hair extension with water from a spray bottle or shower mist. Apply a small amount of the recommended leave-in moisture conditioner and allow the loose extension style to naturally air dry or dry with a diffuser attachment.

For a deep wavy look, do not comb the wave after the hair is dry; for a kinky natural texture, comb the wave after the hair extension is dry. The lace/interlock style can also be wet set or curled with electric curling irons.

To remove your braids

If this is your first time removing your braids, plan two days in advance, in order to time yourself. Longer hair lengths will take more time to remove since you cannot cut the extension that is braided into your hair. Always work in sections so the removal is organized and orderly. After unbraiding at least one quarter of the head, thoroughly comb out that section.

Don't be alarmed if, seemingly, large amounts of your hair comb out. This is a natural process where new hair replaces old hair; pushing the old hair out of the hair follicle. Daily shedding is a natural occurrence that you don't see when the hair is braided. So two months of daily shedding (50-80 strands of hair everyday) is the accumulated hair that combs out once you remove the braids. After each braid removal, your hair needs to be thoroughly combed out, brushed, to stimulate the scalp, shampooed and deep conditioned with a hair and scalp treatment.

Remove synthetic and human hair extensions the same way <u>with one important exception; do not cut the human hair extension</u> if you plan to reuse it.

1. **For synthetic braids, cut below your natural hair and with gentle strokes, unbraid from the bottom up and discard the extension.**
2. **For human hair extensions, <u>do not cut</u>; unbraid from the bottom up. Arrange the extensions in small bundles to be shampooed separately.**

Cleaning human hair extensions for re-use

(Superior quality human hair extensions can be shampooed and re-used.)

1. **Unfold and arrange the hair extensions straight, in four to five bunches. Tie at the center of each bunch.**
2. **Fill a basin with warm water. Pour a small amount of shampoo into the running water.**
3. **Hold a bunch by the tie and dunk it up to 12 times in a basin of warm shampoo water. Rinse the same way in clear water.**
4. **To condition the hair extensions, add condi tioner to lukewarm water and swish the extensions from side to side in the water.**
5. **Rinse in clear water and lay the extensions on a towel to dry. The clean human hair extensions are ready for reuse.**

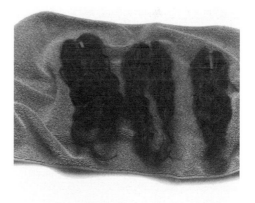

Details to avoid problems with your braid style

Some people believe braids are magical because they make the hair grow, especially the black woman's hair; braid it for a long time and you can be sure to grow a full head of hair. Well, it's not the braids that grow the hair, but the fact that the hair is covered, protected and undisturbed. Curly hair texture has a tendency to grow the fastest when there is less styling, handling and daily combing. The noticeable hair growth, after braiding, is due to not putting heat on it, sponge rolling it, pressing, perming, coloring or applying all the gook from hair sprays, activator, grease, mousses etc.

We know that the average person's hair grows 1/2" per month; so, if it is allowed to do this without the ends being fried and ruined, you will maintain and preserve your hair during normal hair growth. Hair that is braided correctly will show considerable growth; however, if you have experienced hair breakage and balding from braids, you should be aware of several things:

1. Braiding the hair too tightly. Braids should never be unbearably tight and uncomfortable. If during the braiding process you feel pain, a headache or notice the skin pulling where the braid starts, the hair is being pulled too tight. Extreme tightness will cause inflammation, infection or pustules around the part and at the beginning of the braids. Parents are guilty of this too; they braid their child's hair tightly to smooth the edges and to keep the style in for weeks. This is harmful and can cause what is known as Traction Alopecia along the hairline. Traction Alopecia is permanent baldness from pulling the hair out. There is no cure for too tight braids other than removing the uncomfortable braids. The myth that water, oil or time will rid the pain is untrue. If your hair is extremely tight, remove the braid immediately in order to prevent further damage to your hair and scalp.

2. Braiding the hair in the same direction for years, especially around the hairline. The hairline is usually the most fragile and delicate area, so change that off-the-face style occasionally. Constant pressure to the same area can weaken the hair over a long period of time.

3. Poor hygiene. Some women are known to not shampoo their braids for two months in order to preserve the braid style. Having your hair braided more often because of regular shampooing is well worth the investment. A pretty hairdo is not worth an infected, dirty, itchy, flaking scalp. The scalp is an extension of your body, so not shampooing is like not washing your body for months. A filthy scalp can lead to dandruff, dry scalp, head lice and hair falling out.

4. Hair coming out after removal. Don't be alarmed if a lot of your hair combs out after removing the braids. You naturally shed and replace hair daily. Normally you will shed 50-80 strands of hair per day; however, if you are not combing the dead hair out (which is not possible with braids), it will accumulate and comb out in handfuls after

removing the braids. While the hair is in braids, the daily shedding process continues but the hair is not combed out. After several months of not combing out dead hair, you will comb it all out at one time. The only time for concern is if you notice bald spots on the scalp as the hair is shedding.

5. Don't cut hair frizz from the braids after the first day. As the hair grows, your natural hair may frizz through the braids. If you cut this hair frizz, you may be cutting in the middle of the hair strand.

6. If the hair is weak and fragile, you should not attach the heavy extension braids. The weight of the braid and tension may further weaken and break the hair off. Freshly relaxed (8 weeks) or medically thin hair should be braided with precautions or after the hair has strengthened, using small amounts of extension.

7. Extremely fine micro braids. Extension braids that are attached to a few strands of your hair will eventually weaken and break the hair off. The scrubbing friction during the shampoo is irritating to the strands of hair that the extension is braided onto. The friction and handling of these strands will cause your hair to easily tear where the extension is attached.

8. Braids left in the hair longer than two to three months. Hair that is left uncombed for an extended period will begin to tangle and lock. Therefore the new growth hair underneath the braids may mat, making the braid removal and comb-out process tedious and injurious to the hair.

9. Lint collecting at the base of your braids is caused by residue build-up due to poor rinsing after a shampoo or your clothing fabric. Again be selective about the products you use on your hair and the clothes you wear.

10. Severe itching. This condition is common among extension wearers. Cornrow styles are very restrictive to the scalp being able to freely breath. In some cases, where hair is growing fast or the scalp is sensitive to certain cornrow and extension styles, it may irritate the scalp. Try shampooing once a week or changing to an individual braid style.

Follow these easy braid care instructions to prevent the new growth hair from breaking, tangling or matting and to keep your braid style looking fresh and neat.

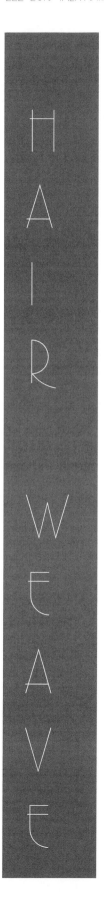

Selecting a weave stylist
Weave and extension styles
Shampoo and grooming

Selecting a Weave Stylist

Natural looking hair weaves reflect a skilled stylist. Many cosmetologists and braiders have jumped on the hair weave band wagon for the sake of money. Their lack of knowledge and expertise, however, has created the bad rap that weave styles get. New methods that are blatantly harmful and not well thought out have caused first-time weave wearers hair loss and embarrassment. Many regret the experience and dislike weaves as a result. It is most important to find a skilled weave stylist who is more interested in protecting and preserving your hair than covering it; a stylist who can cut, style and fashion the hair weave to look as natural and normal as possible. Most importantly, you need a stylist who can take care of your hair so that it grows and thrives beneath the weave extension.

Before having your hair weaved ask yourself, "why am I doing this?" Weaves can be done for fashion, therapeutic and prosthetic reasons -- to grow your hair, to add thickness, to create a style, to add length, to cover a balding area or just because it is a popular style. Once you are clear about why you are weaving your hair, you can easily explain it to your stylist.

Your weave stylist should be patient and take time to consult and discuss with you the style options, home care and the pros and cons. A pre-consultation can prevent last minute decisions and rushed styles that can prove to be disappointing and costly. In advance, consult with the weave stylist so that she may analyze the length, texture, color and condition of your hair. Request to see some photos of her work and samples of the different textures and colors of hair extensions she recommends. This is an important step to be sure your weave stylist has resources for good quality hair extensions and does not expect you to run to the corner store to buy some.

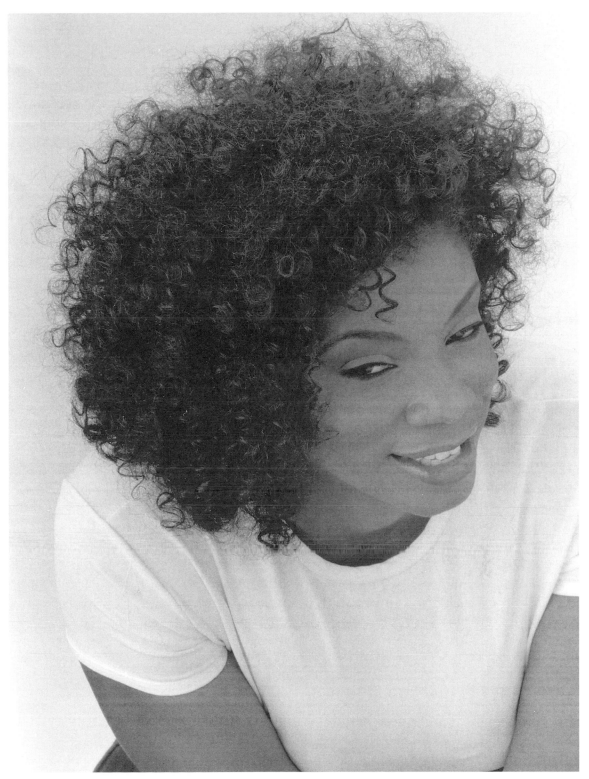

Afro interlock weave

In the consultation, discuss what style you like and any versatility you may want. For example, do you want to pin up your hanging weave style? Do you plan on wearing the weave style towards the face and off the face (this takes pre-planning)? And finally, how will you take care of the weave once you leave the salon? The weave stylist should be able to tell you how to shampoo, style and groom your hair weave at home. If you should decide to go to the salon for maintenance, how often should you go and what will be the cost? What is the expected cost to remove and reweave your style after two months? Be sure to ask what technique and method will be used and how long it will take.

If a braider or stylist seems secretive, defensive or irritated by your inquiries, continue to look for the right weave stylist. Avoid methods that use glue, adhesives, thread wrapping and heat applications. I have found that these methods cause breakage and may cut the hair. They were developed for stylists who do not know how to braid but want to offer weave services. A skilled hair braider can comfortably work with hair as short as one inch on most hair textures. They will also be able to judge if the haircut is too blunt, too fragile or too straight to hold the foundation braid of a weave. The braid weave method is one of the oldest techniques for hair attachments and if done by an expert braider or stylist, will grow the hair and easily last at least two months.

Unless the hair is silky, straight or very short, hair weaves that loosen weekly and need frequent re-tightening may indicate that the stylist does not know what he or she is doing. A knowledgeable stylist will determine, based on the condition of your hair, whether the weave will last the recommended time period. The most important concerns you should have about weaving your hair are that the style looks natural, is easy for you to maintain and is healthy for your hair.

The braid hair weave method can give any woman the length, texture or hair color she may desire. Although the hair weave is used for fashion, it is also a prosthesis hair replacement for women who suffer permanent hair loss. I recommend weaves as an alternative for women who are inclined to chemically texture their hair. You do not have to perm, color or relax your natural hair to wear a hair weave. If given the choice between chemically styling the hair or add-on hair, the hair extension is an overall healthier choice. My concern has always been the unnecessary exposure to (possibly) toxic chemicals on the skin, blindly, for the sake of style.

A hair weave that covers the natural hair, protects it from daily combing and styling. It is a safe way to achieve a different hair color or texture without being permanently locked into that change. Some women will wear a straight texture weave while growing their relaxer out. Even though a woman may choose to wear a Eurocentric weave style, when and if she decides to sport her natural tresses, she can do so by simply removing the weave.

The braid weaving process is painless and quite simple if it is done by a skilled hair braider. The process involves braiding the hair in lines of cornrows and then sewing on wefted extensions. No glues, adhesives, thread wrapping or heat guns are needed by the expert braider. The true expertise is realized in flat braiding, track placement and finishing the style so that it blends perfectly to look like your own hair. If you know someone is wearing a weave, chances are the hair is too long, is wiggy hair and artificial looking. Keep it real and save fantasy looks for the theatre and entertainment business. For example, it will be quite obvious to your family and friends if you walk in with 20 inch, long, blonde, wavy hair; when the day before, you had 3 inches of brown, curly, kinky hair. A realistic weave will save you embarrassment, ridicule and unwanted questions. There is nothing wrong with weaving the hair short to resemble your own hair length so that the change is subtle.

Different Methods to Create Braid Weave Styles

Hair weaves can be partial or full. A partial weave adds hair only where needed. You may need as few as one or two rows, placed, to blend in with your hair. If your hair is short or thin in certain areas, single rows of wefted hair can be added in that area only. The full weave, on the other hand, generally covers 90-100 percent of the hair. It is a style option that allows you to try different cuts, hair colors, textures and styles without affecting your own hair. If your hair is long and you would like to try shorter hair, weave it and cut the weaved hair into a short style. If you always wanted to try a lighter or different hair color than your own, change the hair color with a weave. The true advantage to weave styles is that your hair is protected and you can try many new styles with no obligation.

To create an off-the-face style that looks natural and can be pulled back or up, you will have to leave your hair out around the edges. The technique calls for parting a 1/4 inch hairline and blending it into the extension hair. When using your own hairline, it is important that the color and texture of the extension matches exactly. Although this style of weaving the hair looks the most natural, there are some disadvantages to leaving your hairline out. For example, this style requires daily grooming to blend the two hair textures. The free hairline will not grow as fast as the hair that is braided, since this area will get the most styling and handling. It is more likely to thin and break off. I have seen clients grow 12 inches or more of hair on the interior while the loose hairline breaks off to a length of less than three inches. If this should happen, you will need to alternate between this and a style that braids the entire hairline. A full weave that braids the entire hairline will protect your hairline and preserve the hairs growth. It can also be used to wear an entirely different hair color or to camouflage a balding hairline.

In some cases where the front hairline is damaged and very short, which limits you to an on-the-face style, a full hairline weave braids the total front edge and creates a style that hides the hairline and softly falls to the face. The most common complaint about the full hairline weave is that you cannot pull the hair off the face showing your natural hair edge. If the hair edges are balding, then you definitely would not expose the hair-line. One complaint about braided hairlines is, if the wind blows, it exposes the tracks. These are minor problems that can be resolved by wearing a head band, hairpins or a decorative scarf on windy days. The benefits far outweigh the minor problems of a full hairline weave style may cause. *A weave should take from one to two hours to complete and last at least two months.*

The **Interlock braid** style is very similar to the hair weave because it too, looks like loose-styled hair and its foundation is a cornrow. The difference is how the two techniques are done. The hair weave involves sewing hair onto the cornrow. The Interlock is braided, adding small amounts of bulk hair within the cornrow. Strands of extension hair are braided into the cornrow, giving a loose full effect. With this method, the hair falls with a natural lift and volume. It can be cut shorter than your own hair length, since your hair is in the cornrow on the scalp. Curly textured hair extensions will cover the interlock braids well; however, it is not suggested to use straight hair extensions because the straight texture hair is flat and does not cover the cornrow base. Generally, the Interlock style will last up to eight weeks. The disadvantage is the extension hair may shed, making the style costly to replace after eight weeks wear.

The **Lace braid** is another loose hair braid style. Like the weave and interlock, loose hair covers the braids, but this technique uses the individual braid method rather than the cornrow. Your entire hair length is braided in an individual braid that is covered by the loose extension . With your hair braided throughout the length of the style, you cannot cut it shorter than your hair length. If you are looking for versatility and the ability to pull the hair up into a roll, chignon and pin-up styles, the lace braid is the best choice. To style the hair in an up style with the weave or interlock, you must leave out the hair line or cautiously style the hair, to be sure to cover the cornrows on the scalp. This style, unlike the weave and interlock, can take from eight to twelve hours to braid and after two months wear it can take up to five hours to unbraid .

Some clients will wear a hair weave or extension style for medical and therapeutic reasons. Hair loss, thinning, baldness, and surgical scars are problems that can be safely covered with a beautiful weave style. Women who have been limited by wigs or their own special problems are delighted to find an alternative hair style that feels good and looks natural. The most important objective of the hair weave, in this case, is to be sure the hair that is braided is strong enough to hold the weight of the weave. You do not want to weaken and thin already fragile growing hair.

Questions to Ask in a Pre-Weave Consultation.

1. Request to see photos of weaves that the stylist has done, and samples of the hair extension to be used.

2. How much will the service cost and does that include the hair extension?

3. Have the stylist match your hair color (in good lighting) and texture during the consultation.

4. What is the maintenance and cost to remove and re-weave?

5. How long will the weave last before needing to re-do?

6. Can the stylist assure you it will promote hair growth (not bald areas).

Shampoo and Grooming

Treat the weave hair as you would your own hair; comb it daily, shampoo regularly and don't put a lot of product sprays, gels and grease on the hair. Shampoo as often as normal or at least once a week.

1. Rinse your hair thoroughly under a shower.

2. With shampoo lathered fingertips, massage the scalp in between the weave rows. Work the lathered shampoo through the extension hair lengthwise. (Do not scrub in circular motions.)

3. Rinse thoroughly, apply a rinse out conditioner or if applying a recommended leave-in conditioner towel blot excess water first, then apply a small amount of leave-in conditioner. For rinse out conditioners, after rinsing, towel blot the excess water, comb out with a wide tooth comb and either let the hair air dry for texture, wet set it or blow dry and curl with hot irons.

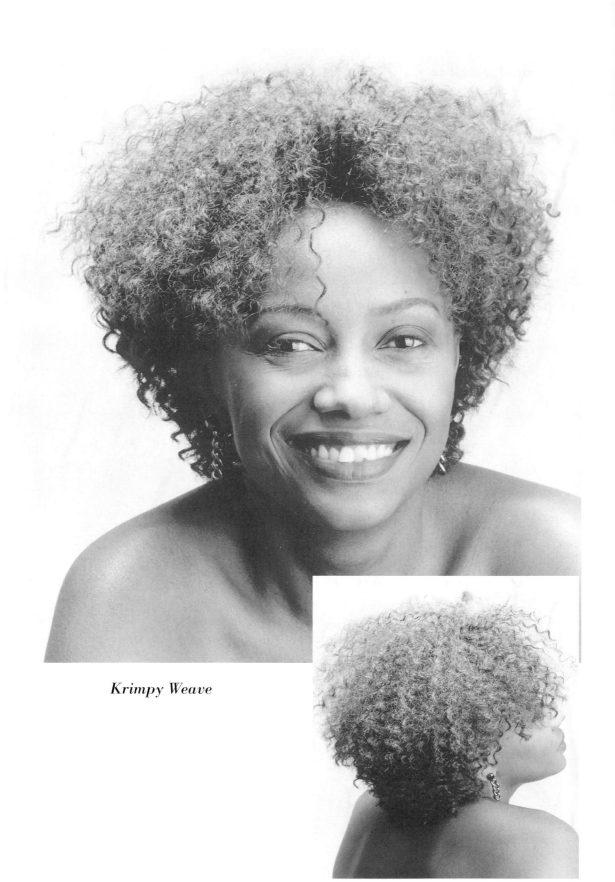

Krimpy Weave

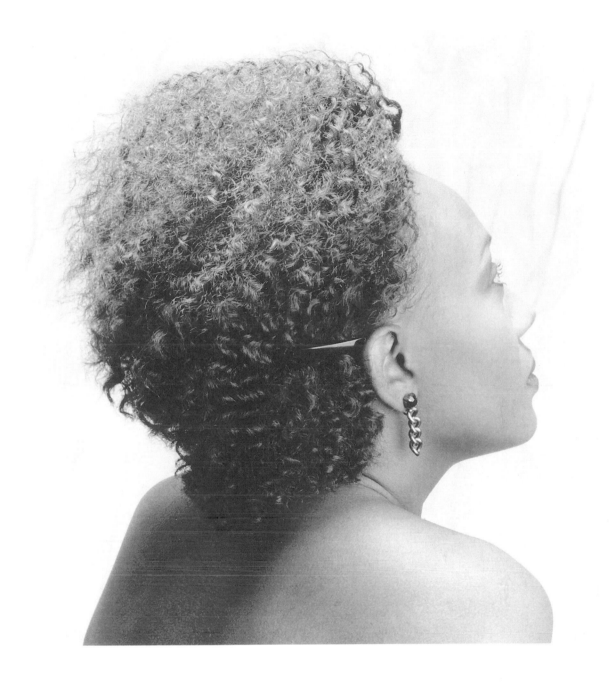

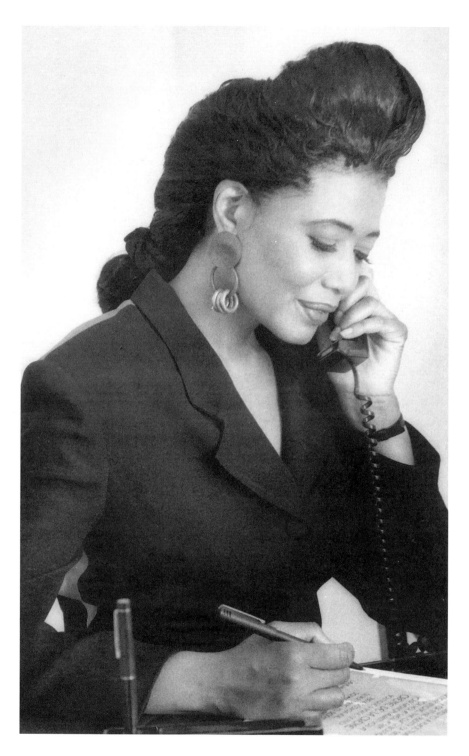

Lace Braids

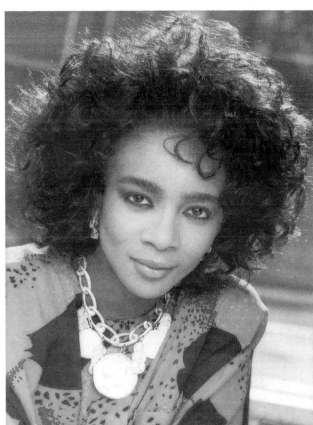

Lace braids

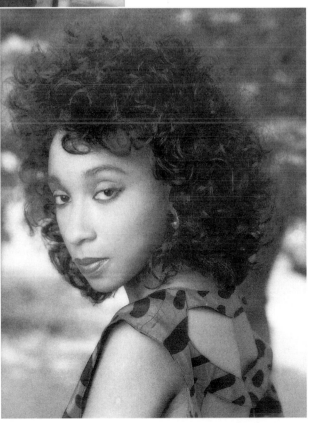

Weave

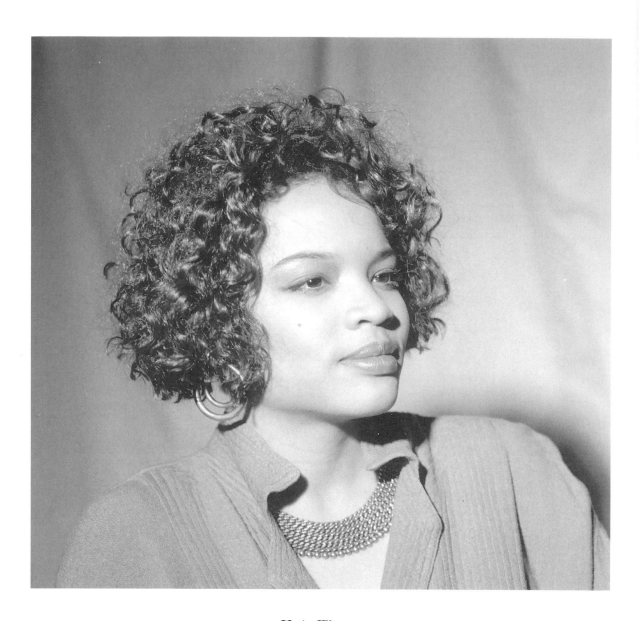

Hair Weave

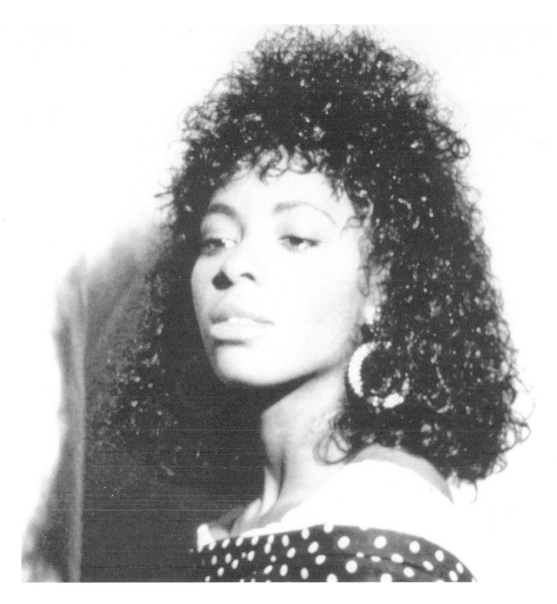

Interlock Braid Weave

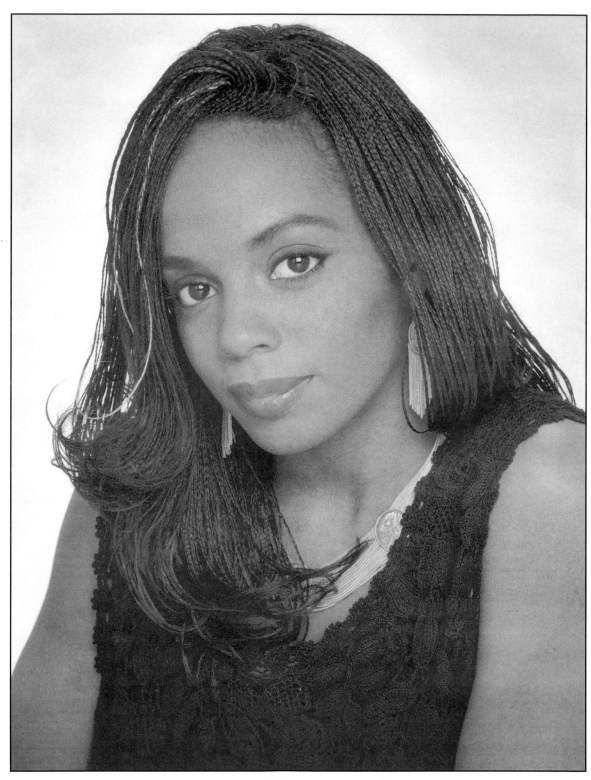

Thousand Braid Weave

Glossary

Braid---three or more pieces of hair interweaved to create a three dimensional section that extends from the head.

Carcinogenic -- the ability to cause cancer.

Cornrow -- a braid pattern that lays flat against the scalp in a row.

Cosmetic -- is a preparation that is formulated to enhance and beautify. It does not claim to treat or heal.

Cosmetologist -- a licensed hair dresser that practices chemical treatments for the hair, european methods of hair styling and beautification practices that are defined by state regulatory laws.

Extensions -- an attachment hair or fiber used to add length, texture or color to hair.

Flat twist -- two pieces of hair criss-crossed to create a rope like pattern that lays flat against the scalp; similar to the cornrow braid.

Hair braider -- a person that beautifies the hair using African inspired styles, natural methods and various techniques of braiding, twisting, cornrowing and weaving of the hair.

Hair Consultation -- to receive advice or be counseled about your hair; how to care for it and be advised about the hair services you may desire.

Handroll -- a hand made curl that is created by winding the hair from the scalp to the ends.

Lace braid -- an individual braid that is covered by a strand of loose hair extension. It gives the illusion of invisible braids.

Locks -- strands of hair that are permanently matted and intermingled to create clusters of hair

Micro braids -- very fine braids that are braided to the end or braided one inch from the scalp and the ends are left loose.

Mutagenic -- the ability to cause damage to the genes and the body's DNA.

Natural hair -- hair that has not been chemically processed in the past two years.

Natural hair care -- to care for natural hair using botanical products that do not permanently change or alter the natural hairs characteristics.

Perm -- a chemical process that makes straight hair curly.

Pin-up style -- a braid or loose hair style that has no hanging ends, like a roll, chignon, invert braid.

Processed hair -- hair that has been chemically colored, straightened, curled or treated with permanently altering cosmetic products.

Relaxer -- a chemical process that makes curly hair permanently straight.

Texturing -- the process of manually twisting, braiding, rolling or shaping the natural hair to have texture. The texture is not permanent; it will only last like a wet set.

Twist -- two pieces of hair criss crossed to create a rope like pattern to the hair.

Virgin hair -- hair that has never been chemically processed.

Weave -- the process of intertwining or attaching loose hair extension to the natural hair. A weave can be achieved using several braid methods.

For more information on these terms see the index.

Bibliography (continued from page 71)

Searle CE, Harnden DG, Venitt S, Gyde OH. Carcinogenicity and mutagenicity tests of some hair colorants and constituents. Nature 1975; 225:506-507.

Garfinkel J, Selvin S, Brown SM. Brief communication: Possible increased risk of lung cancer among beauticians. J Natl Cancer Institute 1977: 58:141-143.

Koeing, K., Pasternack, B.S., and Shore, R.E. (1984) Hair dye use and breast cancer.
Journel of the National Cancer Institute., 71, 481-488
February issue 1979 The Journel of National Cancer Institute.

Ames , Bruce. N., Kammen, H.O., and Yamasaki, E. (1975). Hair dyes are mutagenic: Identification of a variety of mutagenic ingredients.
Proceedings of the National Academy of Science, USA; 72, 2423-2427

Fahmy, M.J. and Fahmy, O.G. (1977). Mutagenicity of hair dye components relative to the carcinogen benzidine in orosophila melanogaster. Mutation Research, 56, 31-38

Footnotes

Page 14/1 Before Freedom Came African-American Life in the Antebellum South,
              The Museum of the Confederacy and the University Press of Virginia. 1991
Page 15/2 Madam C.J. Walker Entrepreneur, A'Lelia Perry Bundles; Chelsea House
              Publishers 1991
Page 17/3 Hair Structure and Chemistry Simplified; A.H.Powitt, B.Sc., ASTC, Milady
              Publishing Corp, NY 1987
Page 54/4 The Consumer's Dictionary of Cosmetic Ingredients, Ruth Winter, Crown Books
Page 58/5 Where Beauty Touches Me; Pamela Ferrell, Cornrows & Co. Publishing
              Washington, DC 1993
Page 59/6 John Peters, MD., et al.; American Journal of Industrial Medicine 3: 169-171
              (September 1982)
Page 59/7 The American Heart Journal; Dec. 1979 Vol., 98; No.6
Page 93/8, 94/9 The Hysterectomy Hoax, Stanley West, MD.; Doubleday Publishing 1994
Page 98/10 Food Healing for Man, Bernard Jensen, Ph. D Bernard Jensen, Publisher;
              Escondido, CA 1983
Page 149/11 Rastafari, A Way of Life; Tracy Nichols, Anchor Press/ Doubleday, NY, 1979

Book References

The Complete Book of Herbs; Lesley Bremness, Viking Studio Books,1988
The New Age Herbalist; Richard Mabey, Collier Books N.Y 1988
Prescription for Nutritional Healing; James F. Balch, MD., Phyllis A. Balch, C.N.C; Avery Publishing Group Inc. NY, 1990
Food Healing for Man; Bernard Jensen, Ph. D, Bernard Jensen, Publisher 1983
Coping with Chemotherapy; Nancy Bruning, Ballentine/Health 1985
The Hysterectomy Hoax; Stanley West, Doubleday N.Y. 1994
The Consumer's Dictionary of Cosmetic Ingredients; Ruth Winter, Crown Books 1984

Special Organizations

**A special thank you to the organizations that have
supported hair freedom and worked with Cornrows & Co.® to fight for
free-enterprise, the right to braid and wear braided or natural hair styles.**

AHNHA
American Hairbraiders & Natural Haircare Association
P.O. Box 9726; Washington, DC 20016-9726
(202) 723-5495, Email: ahnha@aol.com.
*AHNHA was founded to protect the rights of hairbraiders in America and develop standards within the
natural hair care and hairbraiding industry to ensure health and safety standards for the consumer.
AHNHA represents hairbraiders nationwide who challenge state boards of cosmetology about the issue
of hairbraiding. For more information and how you can become a member write or call.*

Eric Steel, Esq.
1119 Twelfth Street., NW; Washington, DC 20005-4632
(202) 842-4794
Attorney Eric Steele is at the forefront of the fight for women discriminated against for wearing braid
styles. He has successfully represented numerous hair discrimination cases on behalf of African-
Americans who filed suits against the Marriott Corp., Hyatt Hotels, American Airlines and numerous
other employers. He also drafted the first hair braiders legislation which became law in Washington, DC.

The Institute for Justice
1717 Pennsylvania Avenue, NW Suite 200
Washington, DC 20006
The Institute for Justice gave definition to Cornrows & Co.'s fight to braid hair. This non-profit public
interest organization fights for free-enterprise and economic liberty; the right of every American to earn
an honest living. Through litigation, the Institute secures protection for individual liberties, property rights
and school choice. Your donations and support of this organization can be sent to the above address.

Photography

The A'lelia Perry Bundles/ Walker Collection; Alexandria, VA (pg. 15)
Hair by Dr. JoAnne Cornwell; Sisterlocks, San Diego, CA (pg. 168-170)
Gillette Research Institute; Gaithersburg, MD 20879 (pg. 72,74)
Pivot Point, <u>Hair</u> <u>Additions</u> (hair by Pamela Ferrell); Chicago, IL (pg. 233)
Kieth Majors Photography; NY, NY (pg 175); Model left /Daphne Crosby
Andre Richardson Photography, Washington, DC
Computer graphics, illustrations & book design; P. Ferrell, Final edit, T.A. Uqdah
Research/ Elizabeth Johnson; Braid Stylist/ Tonya Matthews, Wanda Ferrell

Index

Index

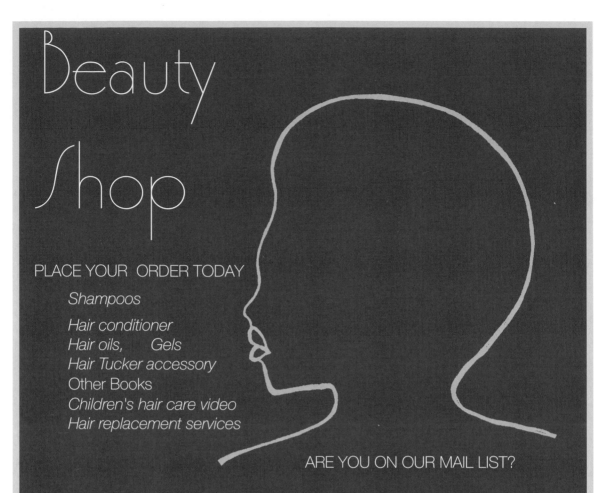